"But I am one of many / And we are strong"

Cancer

Conne

ctions

Credits

Writer: James Burns

Photo Editor: Andrew Stawicki

Designer & Art Director: Paul Haslip/HM&E Design

Junior Designer: Alodie Peñarubia

Production Editor: Pauline Ricablanca

Copy Editor: Eleanor Gasparik

Printer: Friesens Printing Ltd.

John Wiley & Sons Canada, Ltd.

6045 Freemont Blvd.

Mississauga, Ontario L5R 4J3

Printed in Canada

1 2 3 4 5 FP 15 14 13 12 11

Library and Archives Canada Cataloguing in Publication

PhotoSensitive

    Cancer connections: images of hope and courage across Canada / PhotoSensitive.

Based on PhotoSensitive's Cancer connections exhibition.
Issued also in electronic format.

    1. Cancer—Patients—Canada—Pictorial works. 2. Cancer—Canada—Pictorial works. 3. Cancer—Patients—Canada—Biography. 4. Cancer—Canada. 5. Documentary photography—Canada. 6. Black-and-white photography. I. Title.

ISBN 978-0-470-96449-1

TR681.C36P46 2011 779'.9616994 C2010-906497-6

978-0-470-93853-9 (e-PDF);
978-0-470-93852-2 (e-Mobi); 978-0-470-93854-6 (ePub)

Other PhotoSensitive Publications

1995, Precious Time

2000, PhotoSensitive, Ten Years: A work in progress

2005, Life of Water

2007, Vibrant Communities in Focus

2009, Inspiring Possibilities

2010, Field of Vision: PhotoSensitive and social change

Cover

Becky

Becky, a breast cancer survivor, with her daughter and her friends. "My cancer journey taught me how to live, love, and laugh through my family and friends supporting me," she says.

Photographer
Michele Taras
London, Ontario

Foreword

Diane

Diane Courtney was diagnosed with breast cancer in December 2007 at the age of 44. She has undergone a lumpectomy, chemotherapy, and a mastectomy with reconstruction. With the support of her husband (photographer, Michael) and her community, she has strived to keep life as normal as possible for her children.

Photographer
Michael Courtney
Langley, British Columbia

Environmental Benefits Statement

John Wiley & Sons Canada saved the following resources by printing the pages of this book on chlorine free paper made with 10% post-consumer waste.

Trees	Water	Solid Waste	Greenhouse Gases
9 Fully Grown	4,110 Gallons	250 Pounds	853 Pounds

Calculations based on research by Environmental Defense and the Paper Task Force. Manufactured at Friesens Corporation

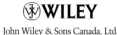

John Wiley & Sons Canada, Ltd.

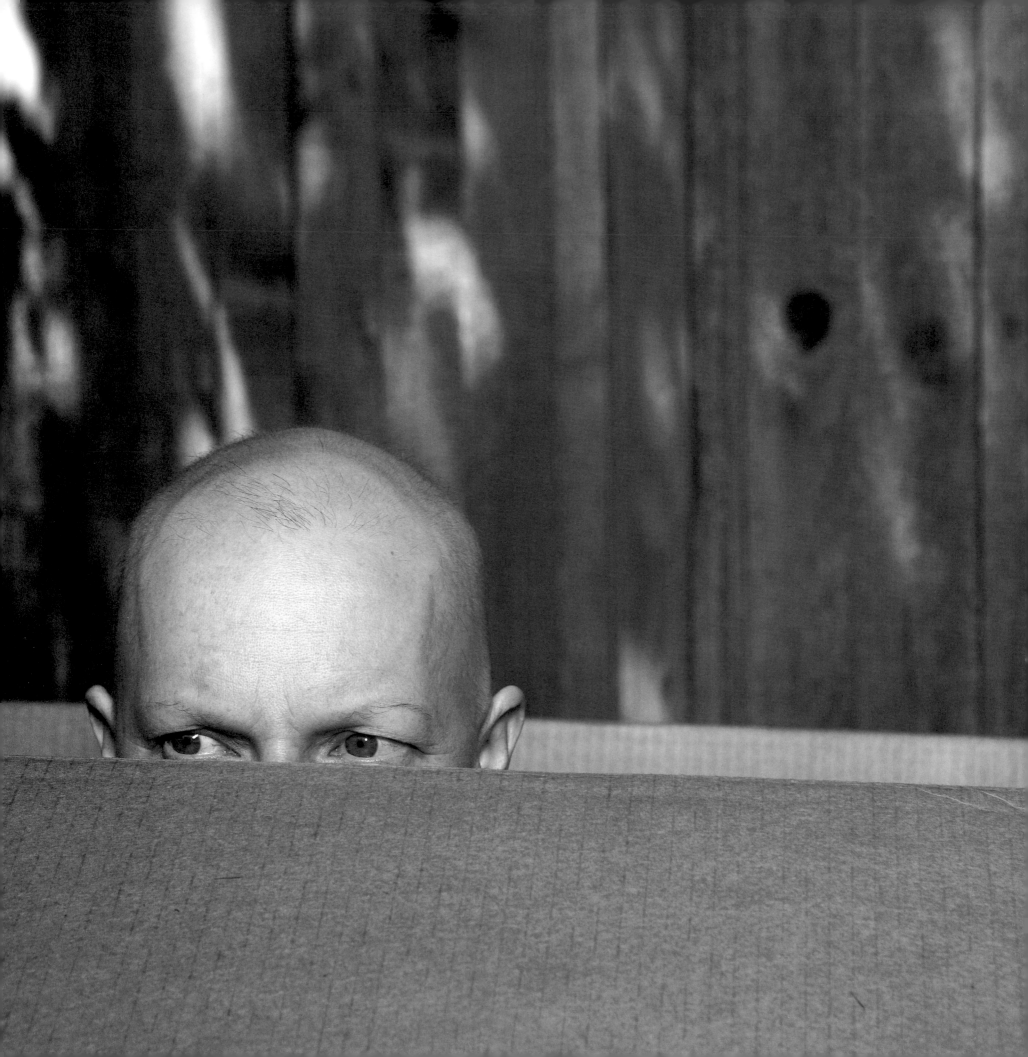

Foreword

The book you are holding in your hands comes from five years of thought and action. What began as a quiet family discussion in Mississauga, Ontario, blossomed—first into a photographic exhibit in Toronto, then into photo exhibits across the country. Along the way, we launched a website and, now, we bring it all together in this book of black-and-white photographs and stories, a celebration of cancer.

Celebrating cancer? It seems to be an oxymoron, and yet that is exactly what this book does: it reveals, it examines, it unfurls a tapestry of what cancer looks like, through the eyes of Canadians who have met it, up close and personal. And the revelation is uplifting and inspiring.

A few years ago, Toronto photographer Andrew Stawicki was watching a TV documentary on cancer with his family. His children prodded, "Daddy, why haven't you done a project on cancer? It's everywhere. You should be doing something!"

Andrew knew they had a point—his photography group, PhotoSensitive, had looked at many difficult issues, from the homeless in downtown Toronto to HIV/AIDS in Africa, but cancer? Where would he start? How could you do justice to something that touches so many people and takes on so many different forms?

But then, on a visit to an elementary school, one of the students asked Andrew what kinds of topics PhotoSensitive tackled. Andrew started by explaining that he believed black-and-white

photographs have a special power—to show the faces of people and reveal their stories. Then he blurted out, "Cancer, for instance. That's a big topic. How many of you know someone with cancer?"

Every child in the classroom put up their hand.

Then they began calling out, "My mom had cancer … My dad did … my brother … my little sister … my grandpa … my neighbour … my hockey coach … my cousin … my teacher …"

That sealed the deal for Andrew. If every child in a classroom knows someone with cancer—well, that is good reason to go forward. At first, it was going to be a project that the photographers at PhotoSensitive would take on. But that changed.

For previous PhotoSensitive projects, we turned to professional photographers for submissions, but because of Andrew's experience with the school children, we decided *Cancer Connections* should be wide open. Anyone could submit a photograph showing their experience with cancer. First, a trickle, then a hundred, then thousands of images came in. Patients, families, friends, neighbours: everyone sent in pictures.

The goal was to have submissions from across the country. We worked with local Canadian Cancer Society offices to put the word out. They did an amazing job, soliciting pictures, booking speakers, suggesting the perfect locations for the outdoor shows, helping us in each city along the way. In the end, photo exhibits were held in Toronto, Charlottetown, Montreal, Regina, Winnipeg, Saint John, Halifax, St. John's, Vancouver, Calgary, and finally, in Ottawa, where we held an incredible, *national* celebration.

Cancer Connections grew far bigger than we had ever envisioned.

Looking back, there were three reasons for that success. First, this was a show made by ordinary Canadians: anyone could send in a photo. Then, these ordinary Canadians sent us extraordinary pictures: they really captured the feeling of people going through cancer. And finally, we held all the exhibits outside, in public places where people would walk by and be caught up in it all. A businessman on his way to work, a student on her way to class, a family on its way to a soccer game. It was accessible to everyone. Beyond that, everyone wanted to share: share their stories, share in other people's stories.

As the project made its way across the country, hundreds of photographs found a home in the exhibits, from PEI to British Columbia. The photographers sent in short, personal stories with their pictures and those became captions. Sometimes the stories would expand into longer, in-depth interviews. Twelve of those are included in this book. And at the heart of it all are the photographs: startling, shocking, memorable, intimate. They will stay with you long after you turn the final page.

There are pictures of bare breasts—one tattooed with a sunflower; young children undergoing chemo; adults with hurting bodies and healing scars; faces full of fatigue, eyes full of hope. In each,

there is a sense of dignity, patience, and courage. When we asked people why they chose to reveal such personal moments of their cancer experience, the answers were as numerous as the photographs submitted.

One person said, "I *wanted* to reveal it. I have to share it so people can understand. So much of cancer is private. So much takes place behind closed doors. If you saw me on the street, you'd never guess I have cancer. These pictures show what we deal with and how we cope and what the face of cancer and the face of love looks like."

And from Keith Branscombe, a survivor of colon cancer, "Taking pictures of cancer did something for me. I took daily pictures of myself and then I shared them. And now, it's in the light of day. It's part of life. Everyone should see it and meet it and not be frightened by it. When I stood beside my photo at the Toronto exhibit, with other people and other people's photos, surrounded by so-called strangers, I realized: we are all connected. We *are* in this together and that feels comforting."

In the beginning we'd hoped, at the end we knew: *Cancer Connections* connected us as Canadians and as human beings, and as a cancer family.

Going through something as potentially devastating or frightening as cancer is a very private thing. And yet here were Canadians, from across the country, revealing themselves or someone they loved through pictures, telling their stories, sharing their pain

"I am going to live my life the way

I always have…"

Harry D. Ashley

and joy. This project gave people places and ways to spend time, see the images, find something that might help them.

As you look through this book, be prepared to be moved. *Cancer Connections* was—and is—an all-inclusive, no-holds-barred revelation of what cancer looks like, through the eyes of those who have experienced it first-hand. We Canadians, often teased for our tendency to shy away from the limelight, have exposed, in beautiful black-and-white portraits, our collective cancer soul—all of its painful scars and bare breasts and shockingly thin bodies and losses combined with faces full of hope and courage and determination and love.

Although the big exhibit photographs are put away, the spirit of *Cancer Connections* lives on, on the website and with this book. Today—and years from now—you can hold this book in your hands and, we hope, be inspired and comforted. If you're told, or someone you know is told, "You have cancer," this will give you strength. You can say, "Look at all the people who looked cancer straight in the eye!"

We dedicated *Cancer Connections* to our friend, writer June Callwood, who was a guiding light for PhotoSensitive. She was in Princess Margaret Hospital, fighting cancer, when we began *Cancer Connections*, and she told Andrew, "Go for it. It's high time someone did something really inspired." She believed in helping others and making connections and we think she would have been pleased with the scope and spirit of this project.

Through the contribution of countless "ordinary" Canadians, we have created an extraordinary canvas of cancer. *Cancer Connections* celebrates the human spirit and all it can accomplish even when dealing with—and perhaps often *because of*—great challenges, and the love that so often accompanies loss. At the Montreal exhibit, Andrew saw a woman weeping quietly, sitting alone on the grass. When she stopped crying and looked up and spotted him, he walked over and extended a hand, introducing himself.

"Thank you," she said simply. "Thank you. I thought my mother had died but her photograph is here—a wonderful black-and-white portrait of my mother is *here*. She is still alive."

Alive and with a story to tell.

PhotoSensitive
Toronto, 2011

A message from the Canadian Cancer Society

Over a period of two years, Canadians shared their cancer stories as *Cancer Connections* travelled across the country. In that short period of time, the exhibit grew from 300 images to the goal of 1,000 photos. Each image featured in the exhibit represents thousands of similar cancer stories.

As we set out on this partnership with PhotoSensitive, our hope was that *Cancer Connections* would encourage Canadians from coast to coast, in small and large communities alike, to have conversations about cancer. We believe that through sharing cancer stories, Canadians can learn more about cancer risk factors and what they can do to prevent the disease.

Cancer Connections has given Canadians a forum to share how this disease has changed their lives and has provided a unique, accessible way to bring people, communities, and the nation together.

These inspirational black-and-white photographs connect us as individuals and communities in the common cause to fight back against cancer. Through these stories, we see the pain, the frustration, and the challenges that cancer brings, but also the courage, the resolve, the hope, and even the joy that people bring to cancer.

The Canadian Cancer Society firmly believes that no one should face a cancer journey alone. Each year we connect with and support tens of thousands of cancer patients on their journeys.

We are only able to deliver such support through the dedication of our volunteers and staff and the generosity of our donors. They are making "cancer connections" each and every day.

On behalf of the Canadian Cancer Society's volunteers and staff from coast to coast to coast, I thank all those who allowed their personal stories to be captured in *Cancer Connections*. I also want to congratulate the photographers for their skill in showing us cancer through a different lens. Collectively these images are a testimony to the power of photography to address social issues. Thank you to PhotoSensitive for your vision in creating this unique exhibit, and for raising awareness about cancer and how it affects the lives of Canadians. It has been a privilege to partner with you on this truly moving exhibit.

Peter Goodhand, President and CEO
Canadian Cancer Society

Canadian   Société
Cancer   canadienne
Society   du cancer

A message from JPMorgan Chase

As JPMorgan Chase has evolved into one of the world's largest and most influential global financial institutions, our firm's unwavering commitment to making a positive difference in the communities where we operate has remained constant.

JPMorgan Chase's philanthropic goal is simple—be the catalyst to meaningful, positive, and sustainable change within communities across the globe. In 2009, JPMorgan Chase gave more than $100 million through grants and sponsorships to thousands of not-for-profit organizations around the world. Our employees participate in *Relay For Life* events across the country and we support them through the Matching Gift and volunteer programs.

JPMorgan Chase believes in the fight against cancer. We don't see ourselves as merely a supporter of the cause, but rather a partner in this battle. Through thoughts, actions, words, and donations, JPMorgan Chase employees walk arm in arm with the focused objective of beating cancer.

We appreciate the tremendous effort that PhotoSensitive and the Canadian Cancer Society put into bringing *Cancer Connections* to life through photography. The awareness that *Cancer Connections* brought is instrumental in generating ongoing momentum around this cause. The photography and, more importantly, the stories that these images tell are beautiful and inspirational to all Canadians.

So many Canadians, including JPMorgan Chase employees, have to fight this disease every day. With more than 1,000 employees in Canada, JPMorgan Chase has a vested interest in bringing positive change within the communities where our employees live and work. We are fortunate to work with the Canadian Cancer Society and PhotoSensitive, and through our support of Cancer Connections, help to bring a poignant photographic exhibit of those affected by cancer and their families to cities across Canada and now in this book.

We wish the Canadian Cancer Society continued success in fighting cancer, enhancing the quality of life of those living with cancer, and celebrating survivors.

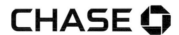

Andrew Pilkington, President and CEO
Chase Card Services Canada

CHASE ⬡

British Columbia

"Many gifts came with my cancer. So much love came at me, so many opportunities."

Nancy Baye

Photographer
Andy Clark
Vancouver

Nancy

When PhotoSensitive arranged for Nancy Baye to be photographed by Andy Clark for *Cancer Connections*, Nancy already knew how she wanted to be portrayed. "I wanted to be photographed breaking out of my hospital gown," she says, "breaking free of the cancer-patient identity and unleashing my inner superhero."

After being diagnosed with breast cancer, Nancy's hospital gown also became the cape for her alter ego, the Cancer Crusader.

"After immersing myself in the cancer community, I witnessed the diversity and range of emotional and sociological issues behind cancer," says Nancy. As a writer and performer, it wasn't long before those observations drove her to pick up a pen. "These different snippets of stories would arrange themselves into a character that suddenly 'showed up' in my mind, a character with something to say."

Nancy wrote monologues for the characters and they in turn were incorporated into performances that she used to open the door to the world of cancer. "This allowed for a multitude of stories and perspectives to be explored, more than could be done in a personal speech. It also provided a buffer to give the audience a sense of safety so they wouldn't censor their responses.

"I wanted them to feel free to laugh as well as cry. The goal was to take them along on each character's journey in a highly experiential, visceral way. Through it all, I wanted to give voice to cancer patients, so that they might be better understood and seen in all their complexities. My hope was that the shows would enlighten and empower while they entertained."

Nancy's shows, including the *Support Group Monologue* and the *Adventures in Breast Cancer* trilogy, have appeared at theatres and fundraising events across Canada.

Having fought breast cancer three times, Nancy has drawn much from her own experiences to bring a truth to her characters. She has been cancer-free since 2004, but takes nothing for granted.

"I felt an ache in my hip recently and thought, 'Oh, my God, it's gone to the bone—I'll be dead within a week,'" says Nancy. "Any little ache or pain has me worried, but doctors watch me closely and I am fine. Knock on wood."

Apart from providing artistic inspiration, Nancy's cancer experiences also provided other positives: "Many gifts came with my cancer. So much love came at me, so many opportunities, I just had to be willing to accept it all and not resist the journey. Cancer has matured me in many ways and it has also allowed me to take flight. I believe that cancer can bring out the superhero in us all."

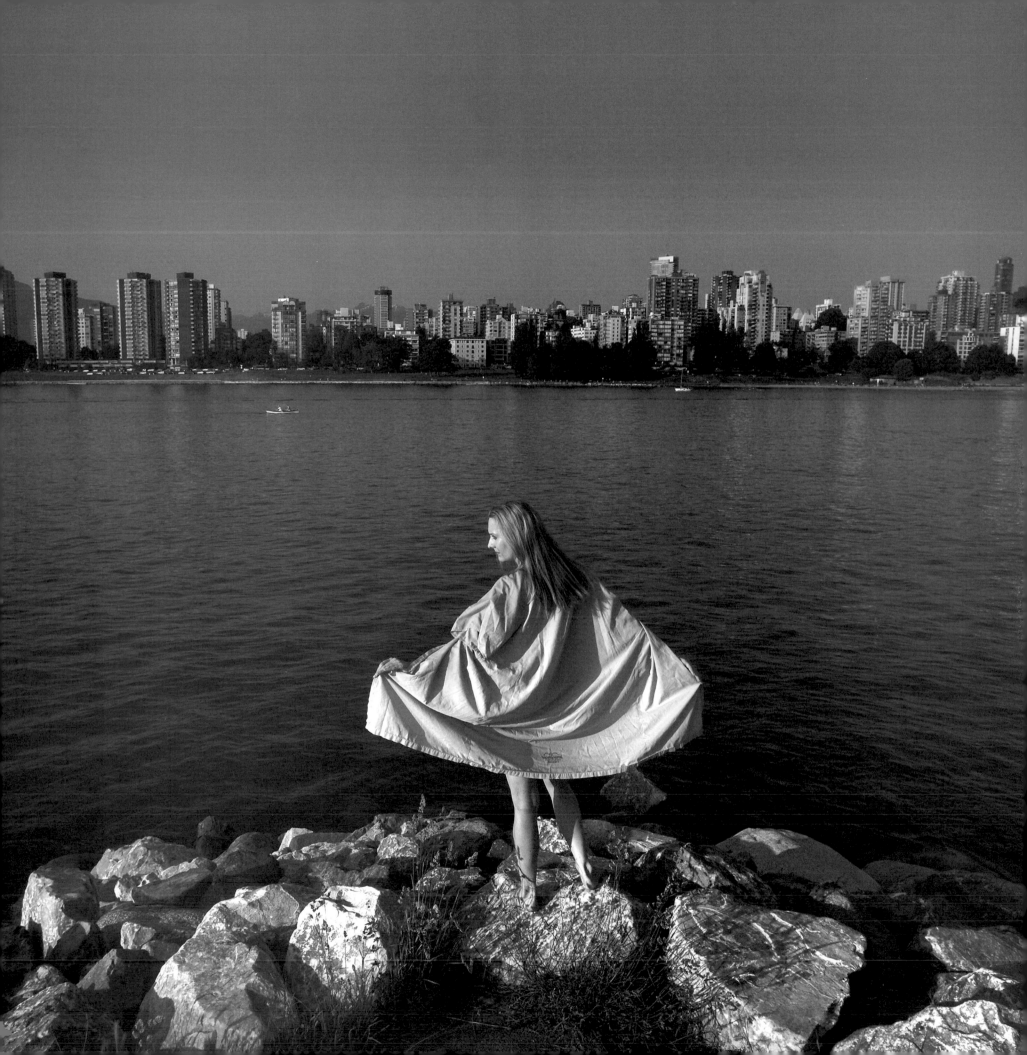

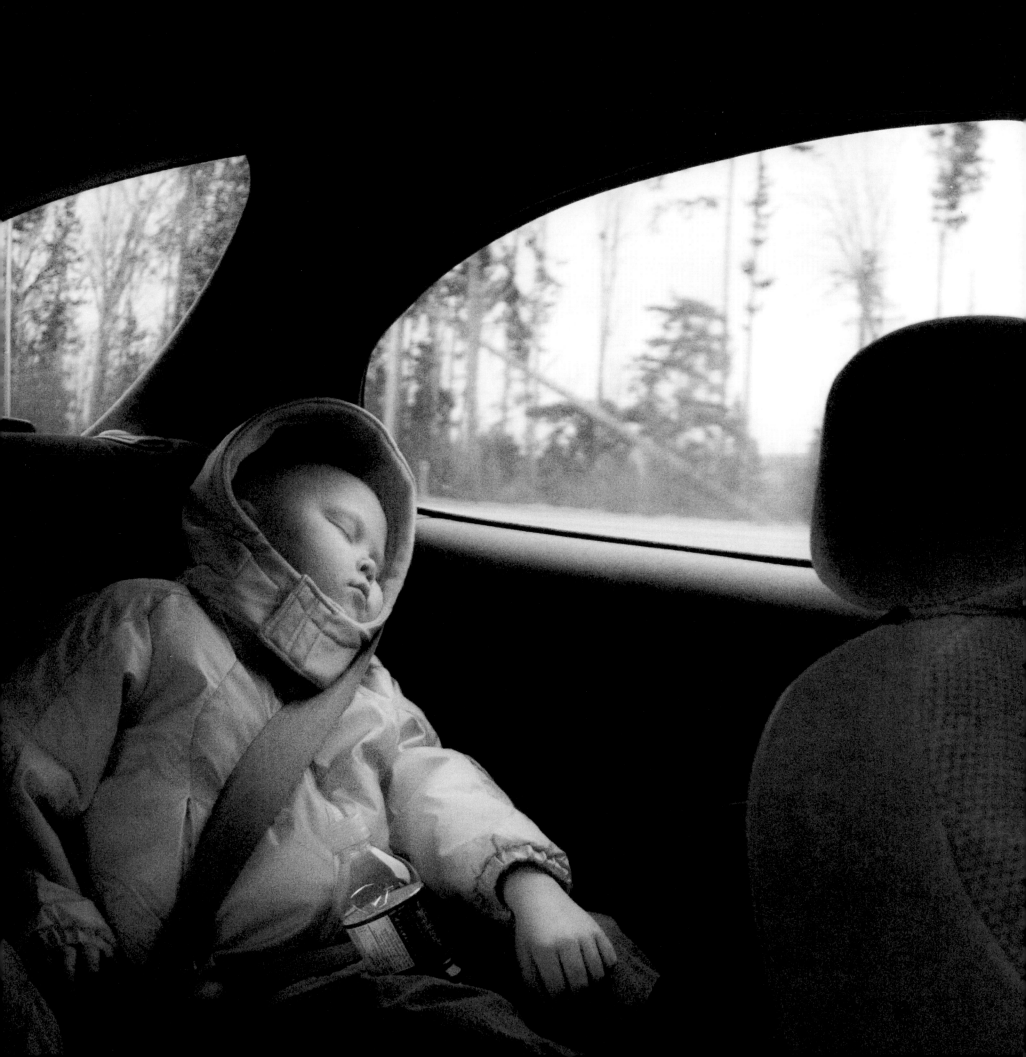

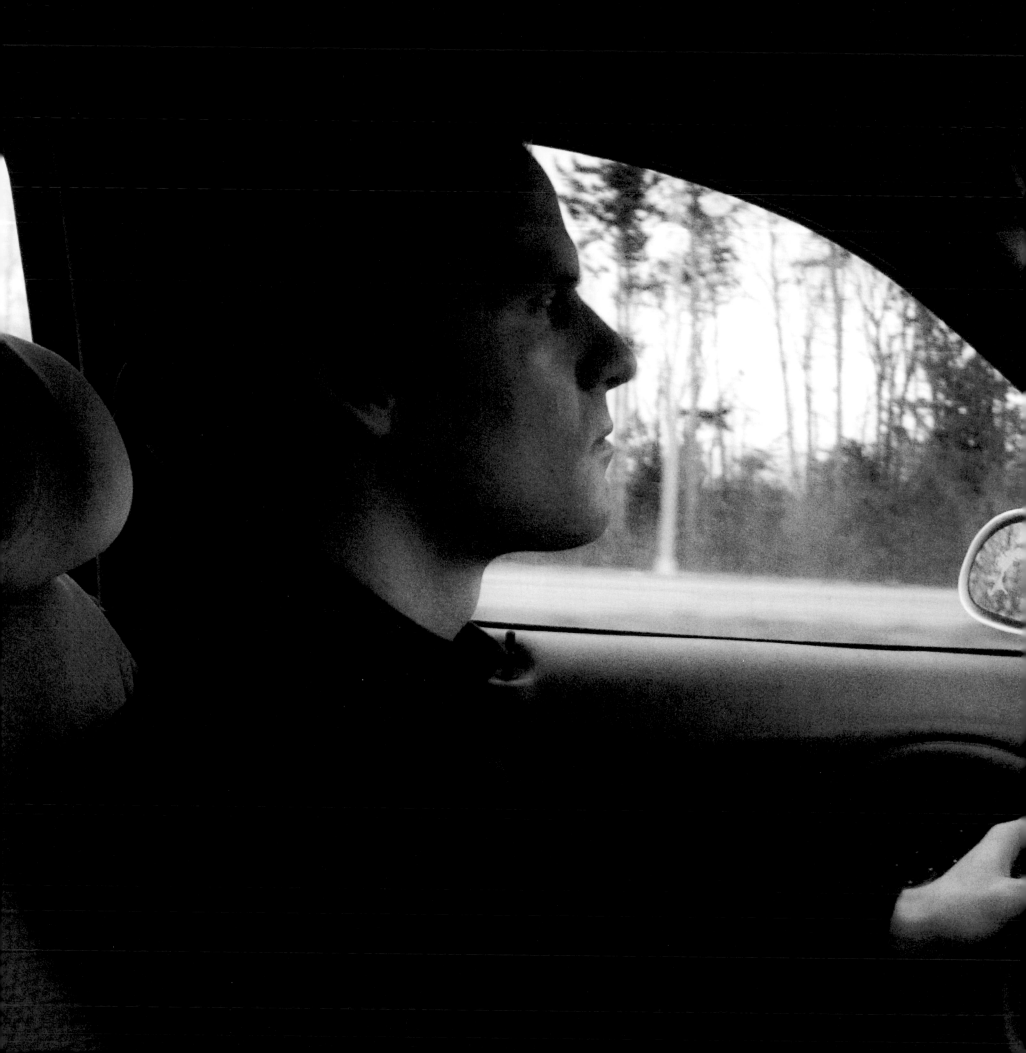

Previous

Maggie

John Johnson driving his young daughter Maggie on the eight-hour roundtrip required for her to receive her leukemia treatment.

Photographer
Karen McKinnon
Comox

Donald

"I am one face of cancer / I am one body scarred by cancer / I am one survivor of cancer / But I am one of many / And we are strong." Donald Golob was diagnosed with stage 3-4 kidney cancer in 2005. After surgery, it came back twice but further surgery removed it. Donald says, "It looks like I just may make it."

Photographer
Tamara Roberts
North Vancouver

Rich

Inspired to action after his 26-year-old, non-smoking friend was diagnosed with throat and lung cancer, Rich Ralph set out to inline skate from St. John's, Newfoundland, to Victoria, B.C. Four months and 10,000 kilometres later, he completed his trip, raising awareness and $60,000 from personal donations collected along the way.

Photographer
Kyler Storm
Vancouver

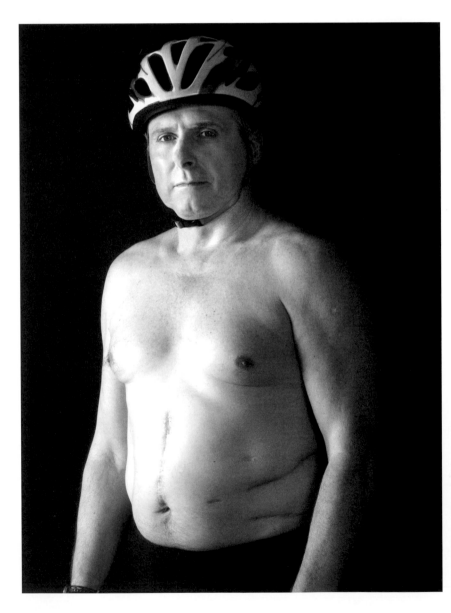

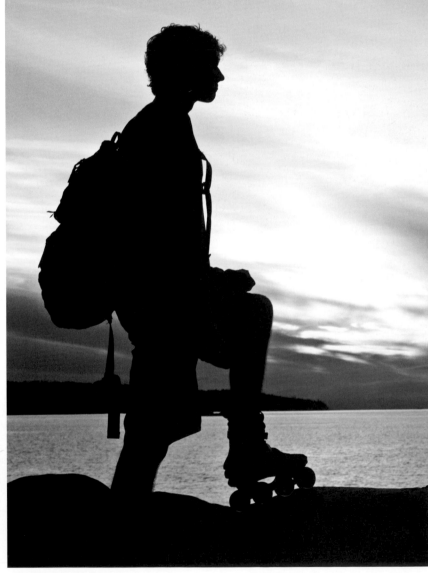

Dragon Divas

The "Cowichan Valley Dragon Divas" team is made up of over 40 members, all living with breast cancer.

Photographer
Paul Fletcher
Duncan

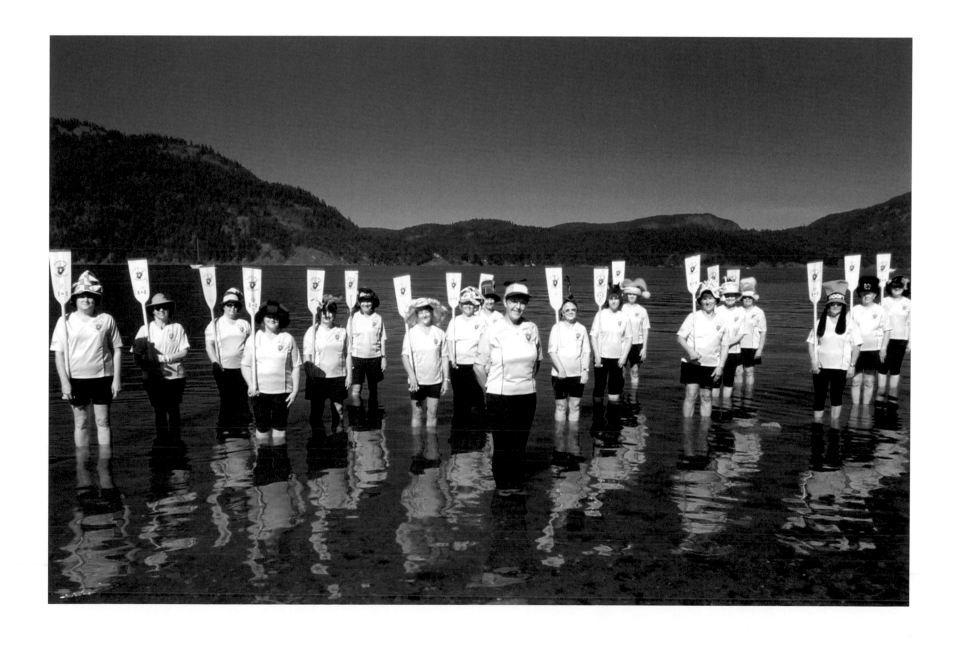

Julie

A self-portrait of the photographer lying on her mother's grave in Chilliwack, B.C. Jennifer's mother died of breast cancer in 2007 and Jennifer herself survived bone cancer as a child. She is lying with the operation scar on her left hip facing the sky.

Photographer
Jennifer Neal
Chilliwack

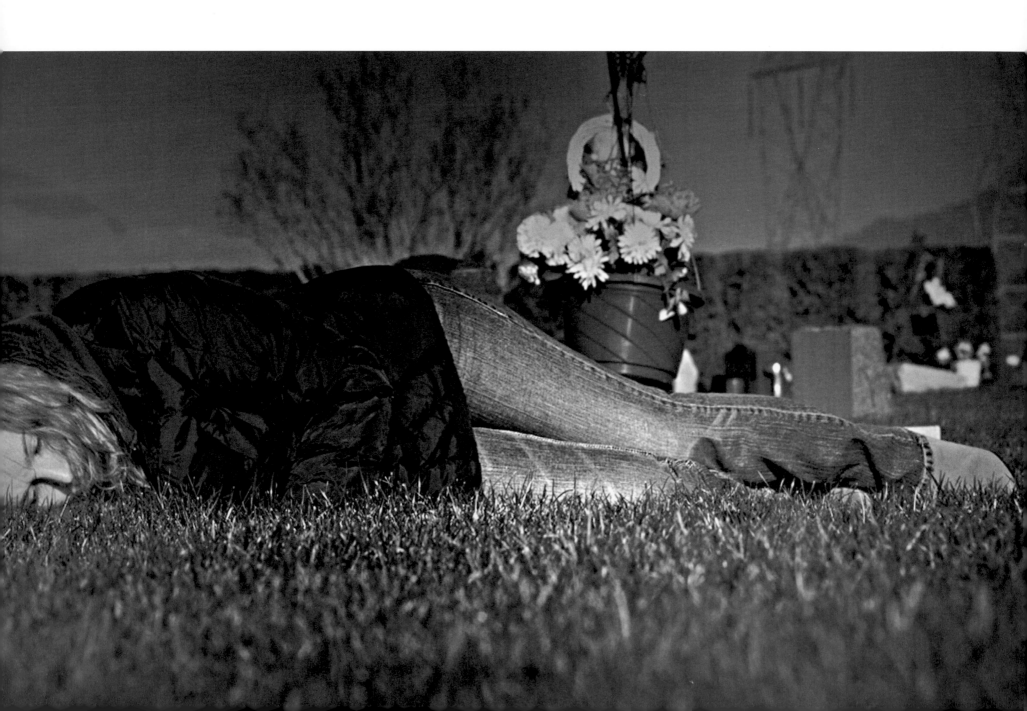

"Never lose sight of even the smallest

things that bring you joy."

Sandra Beuker

Scott

Scott Mitchell, a native
of White Rock, B.C., died
of cancer when he was only
23 years old. Photographer
Laura Sumpter says, "His
dad's vest is a sad reminder
that cancer chooses all ages.
It does not discriminate."

Photographer
Laura Sumpter
White Rock

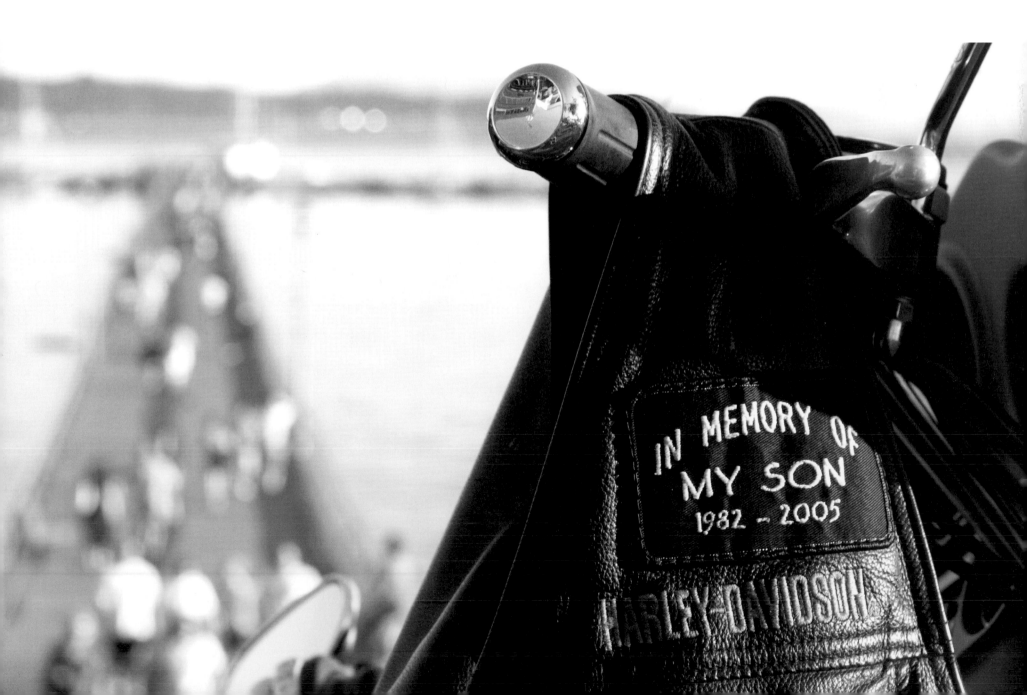

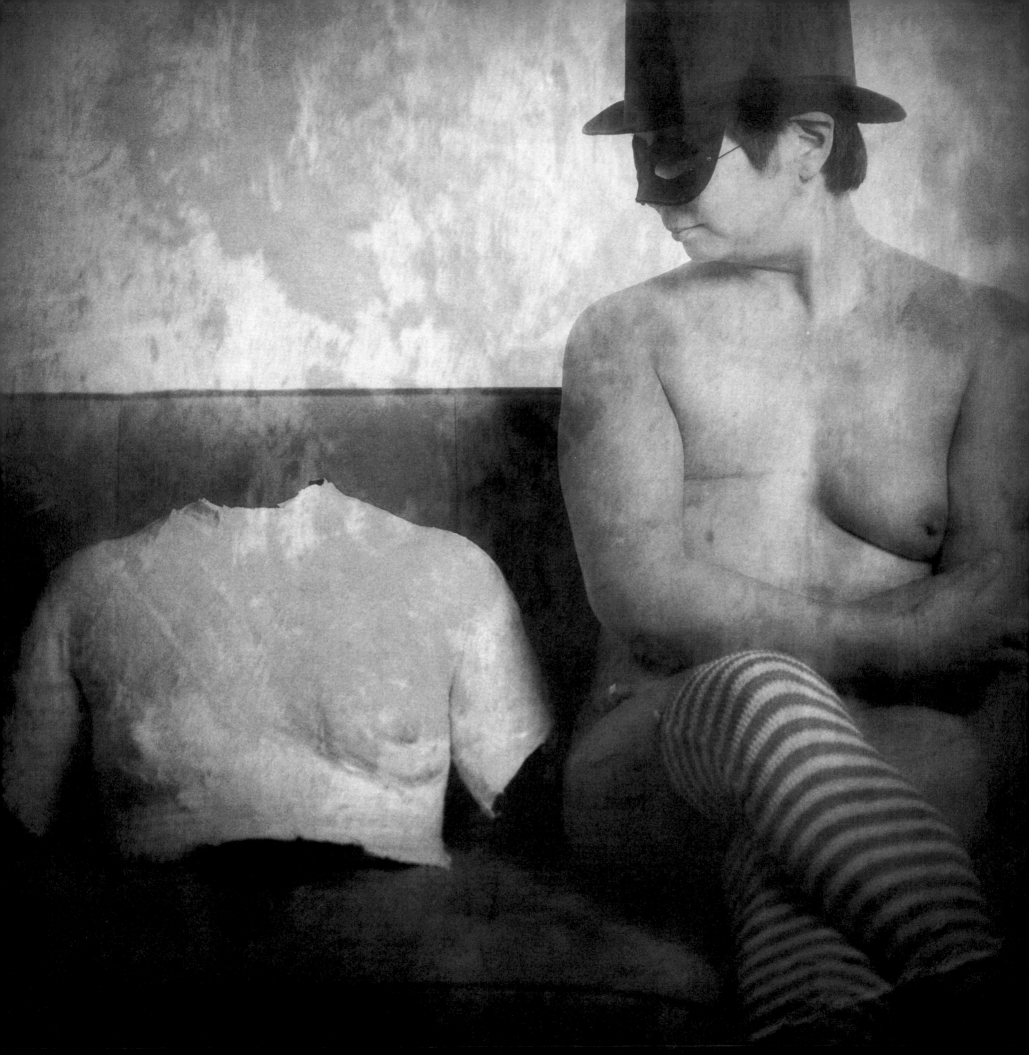

Opposite

A Woman

Post-mastectomy, a woman contemplates the cast she made of her torso before surgery. The mask reflects how the surgery and her breast cancer make her feel like a circus freak. She opted out of reconstructive surgery to act as a role model for other breast cancer survivors. She has been cancer-free for 10 years.

Photographer
Jane Eaton Hamilton
Vancouver

Janelle

After being diagnosed with breast cancer in 2006, starting chemotherapy and realizing she was going to lose her hair, Janelle Hughes sought alternatives to bandannas, hats, and wigs. She created Bald is Beautiful, custom head-dresses and airbrush artistry for women who have lost their hair to cancer. Sadly, Janelle passed away in spring 2008.

Photographer
Carmine Marinelli
Surrey

Rosanne

This self-portrait was shot as the photographer, Rosanne Patricia Currie, was undergoing chemotherapy in preparation for a stem cell transplant. She is still in recovery.

Photographer
Rosanne Currie
Victoria

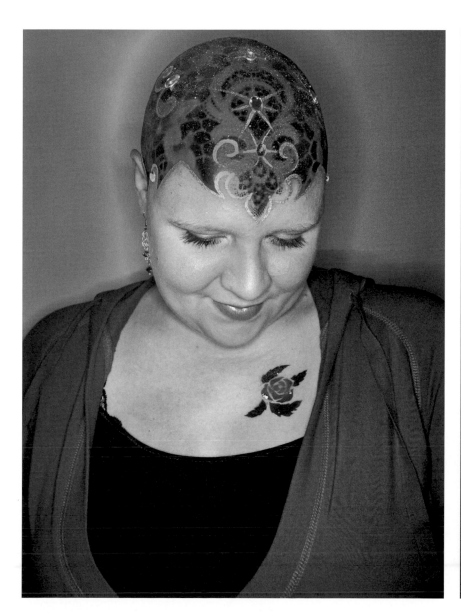

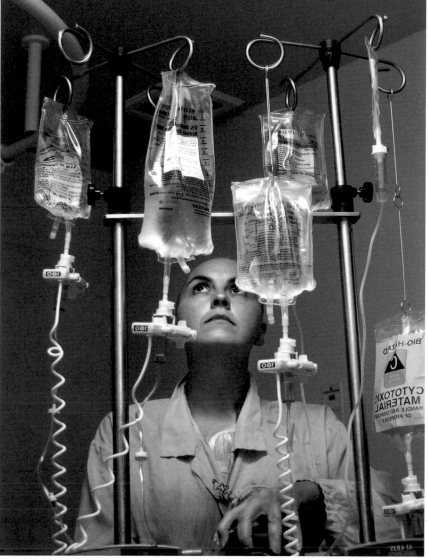

Photographer
Daniel Sikorskyi
Victoria

Daniel

When Daniel Sikorskyi told his doctor that he was having trouble urinating and getting up to pee three or four times a night, he was given a prescription to help him retain urine. Later, Daniel told a chiropractor friend about his symptoms and she pushed him into going for an immediate checkup.

That doctor referred him to a urologist, whom Daniel saw a week later. "I think the urologist had a hunch," says Daniel. "He booked me for a biopsy straight away—which was like having a staple gun shot up your ass. I wouldn't wish that on anyone. After this whole experience I realized there was no room for embarrassment."

A call from his doctor a few days later telling Daniel he had prostate cancer came as a complete shock. "I couldn't believe it. I hadn't turned 50 yet. It took a while to collect myself and think about it. Then I started researching."

Determined to take control of his cancer, Daniel did extensive research, spending hours reading up on the subject. He went on a raw food diet, exercised regularly, had acupuncture, and kept a positive attitude. He also changed urologists, going to one recommended by another of his acupuncturist's clients, who had also battled prostate cancer.

"Dr. Martin Gleave treated me like a human being who had a problem. He was there to help and he took me through the whole process, suggesting treatment but ultimately leaving the final decision up to me."

After much deliberation, Daniel decided to have a radical prostatectomy, an operation that he felt was more likely to rid him of all of the cancer in one fell swoop. "It all went really well," he recalls. "There was some pain involved and things to deal with, but there were no signs of it spreading, so I was happy with that.

"I feel better now than I did before the cancer. My thought processes have changed and become more positive. With cancer, people often wonder, 'Why did it happen?' I believe it happened to enlighten me."

Daniel is now a fervent advocate for prostate cancer awareness and constantly reminds his friends to go for checkups. "They often tell me that they don't like the idea of going for a rectal exam, so I tell them that I don't like the idea of going to their funeral."

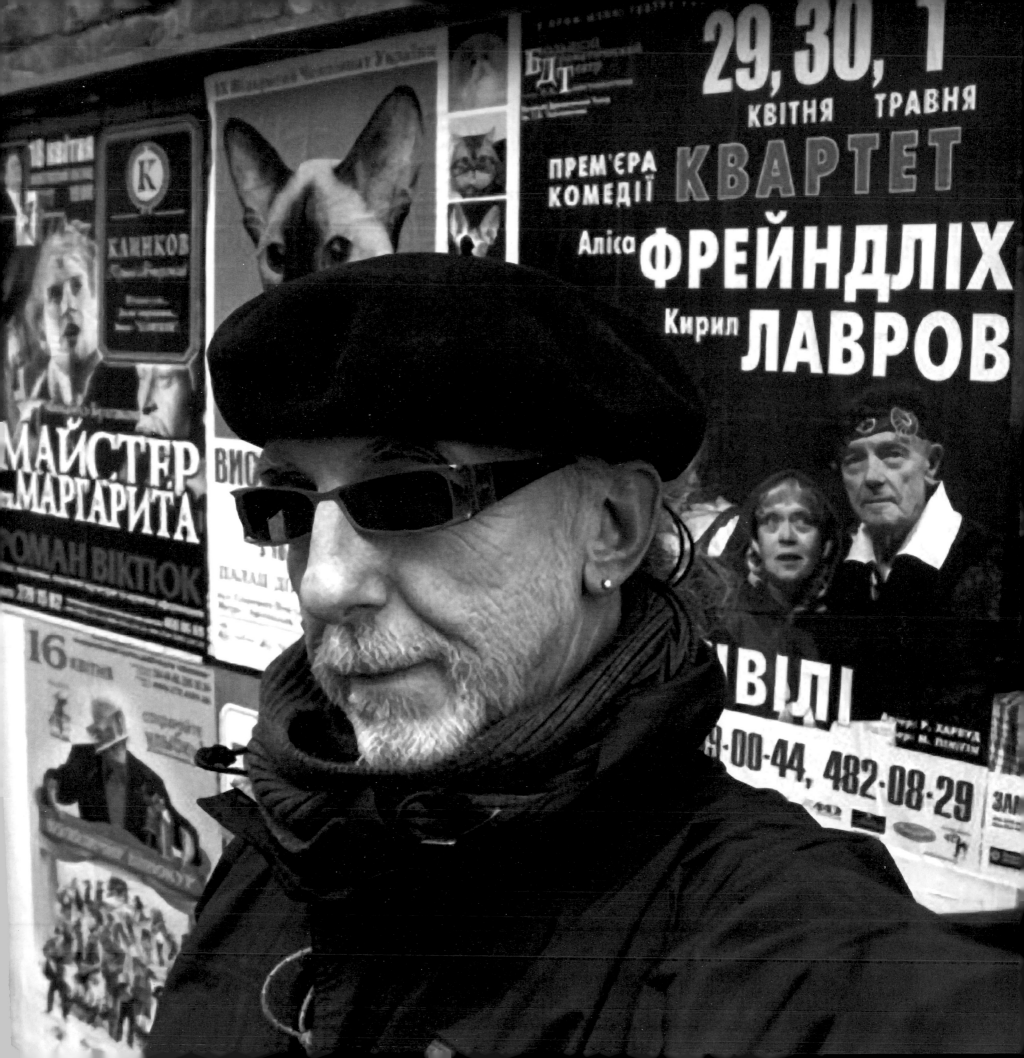

Elly

Elly Ruge's adventure with breast cancer began in 2001. Operations and chemotherapy left her feeling both physically and emotionally scarred. She had a sunflower tattooed onto her new left breast and it has given her a positive attitude to live her life with boundless energy. She hopes to inspire others to see that their scars also can become works of art.

Photographer
Marcelle Ridley
Duncan

Vanessa

After being diagnosed with breast cancer, Vanessa became passionate about promoting breast health awareness for young women and the unique issues that face them. This photo appeared in the 2005 *Breast of Canada* fundraising calendar. Now moving on with her life, Vanessa no longer defines herself as having had cancer.

Photographer
Kimberly Mara
Surrey

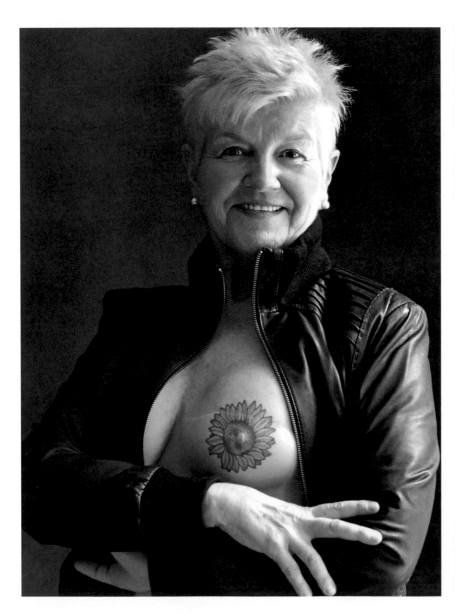

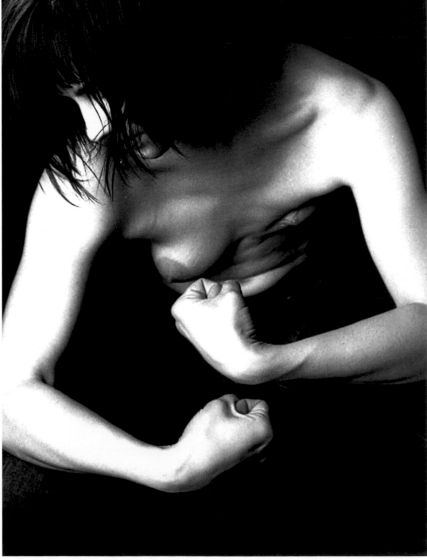

Janet

Janet Winbourne, ethno-
biologist and world
traveller, is a two-time
survivor—of cervical cancer
in 2002 and breast cancer
in 2006. This photo
was taken after she'd had
a partial mastectomy, lymph
node removal, and six
months of chemotherapy.
The following day Janet
started five weeks of radiation
treatment.

Photographer
Sheri Jackson
Port Alberni

Kim

This photo was taken while
Kim Tempest was going
through chemotherapy for
breast cancer. Additional
images taken during her
treatment will be included
in her book, about fighting
breast cancer with humour,
entitled *My Right Tit*.

Photographer
Wendy D
Vancouver

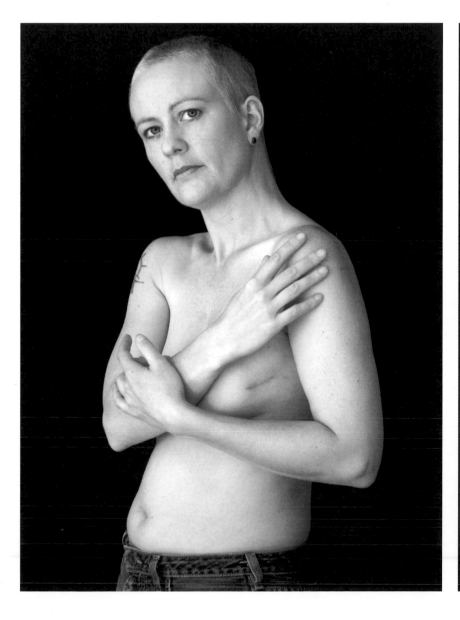

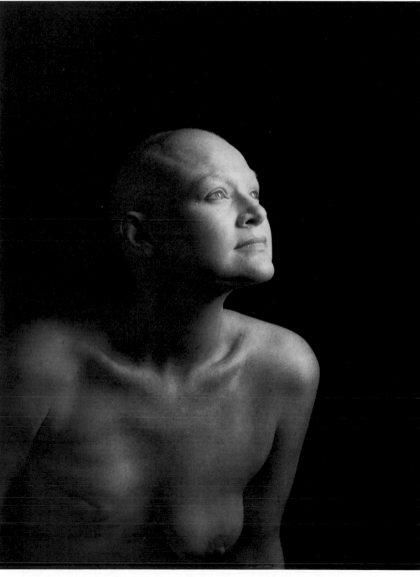

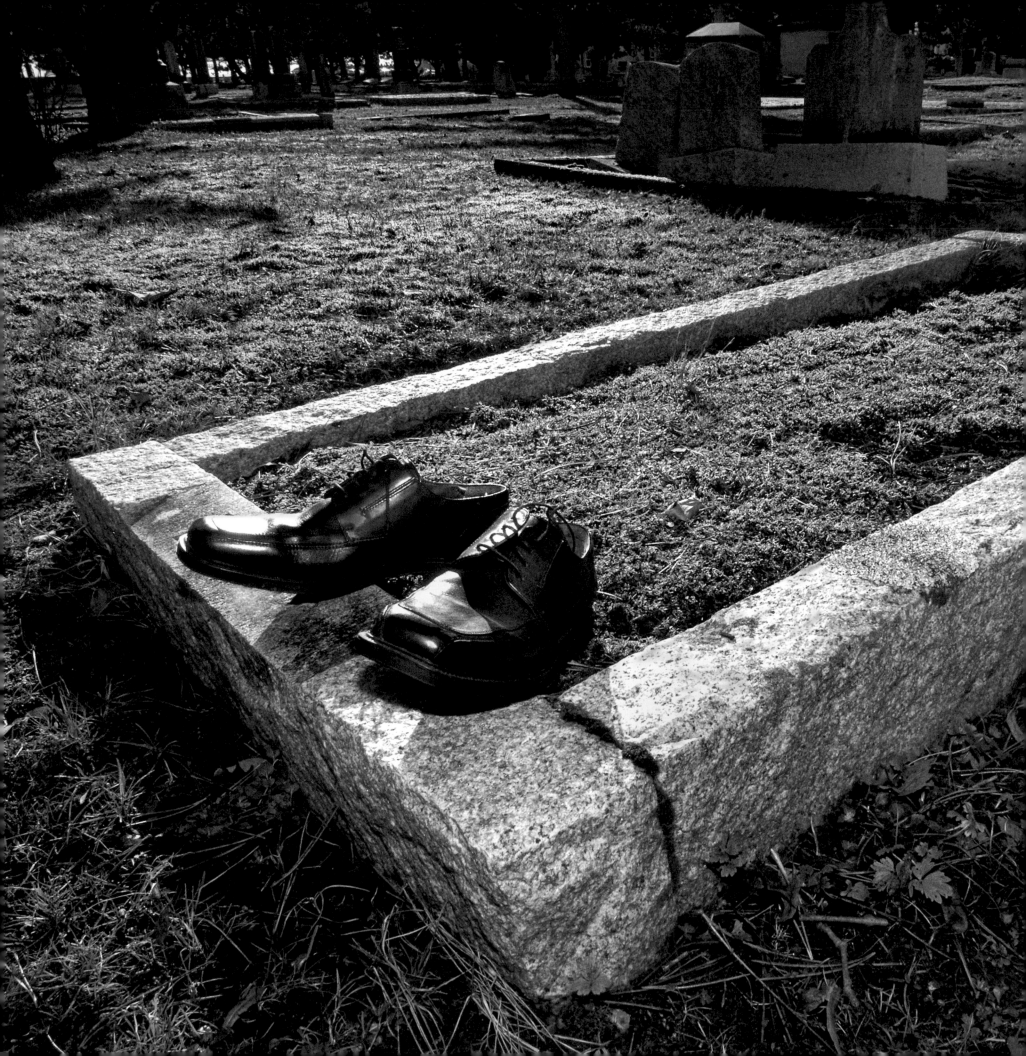

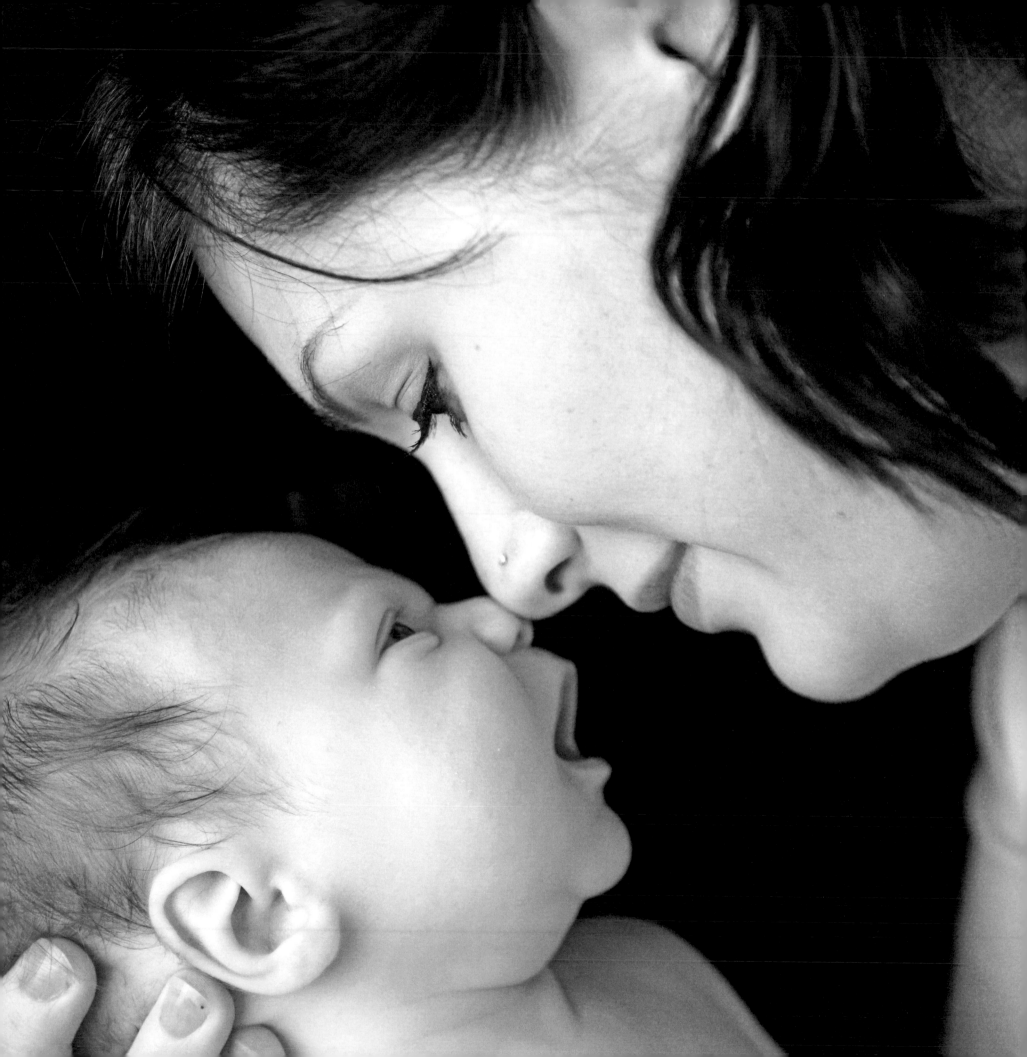

Previous left

Jack

Photographer Alexis was inspired to take this photo in memory of her late husband, Jack Sullivan, who passed away in 1994, after a courageous fight with nasal pharyngeal carcinoma. Alexis says, "I wanted to say that he continues to be so real to us, he might still need his shoes."

Photographer
Alexis Yobbagy
Victoria

Previous right

Lisa

Lisa Matlock used tanning beds in her teens and was diagnosed with melanoma first at age 23, and then six years later when pregnant with her first child. She and her husband were devastated to learn that the cancer could pass to the baby, but thankfully Beckett was born perfectly healthy. Lisa's fight will never be over and she speaks out against the risks of UV exposure.

Photographer
Tanzyn Ambrose
Port Coquitlam

Sandra

The day of Sandra Beuker's final chemotherapy session for breast cancer. Russell, her husband and the photographer, says, "Her grace, strength, and beauty throughout her ordeal inspires me to this day." After chemotherapy, surgery, and radiation, Sandra is doing well. She says, "Never lose sight of even the smallest things that bring you joy."

Photographer
Russell Beuker
Richmond

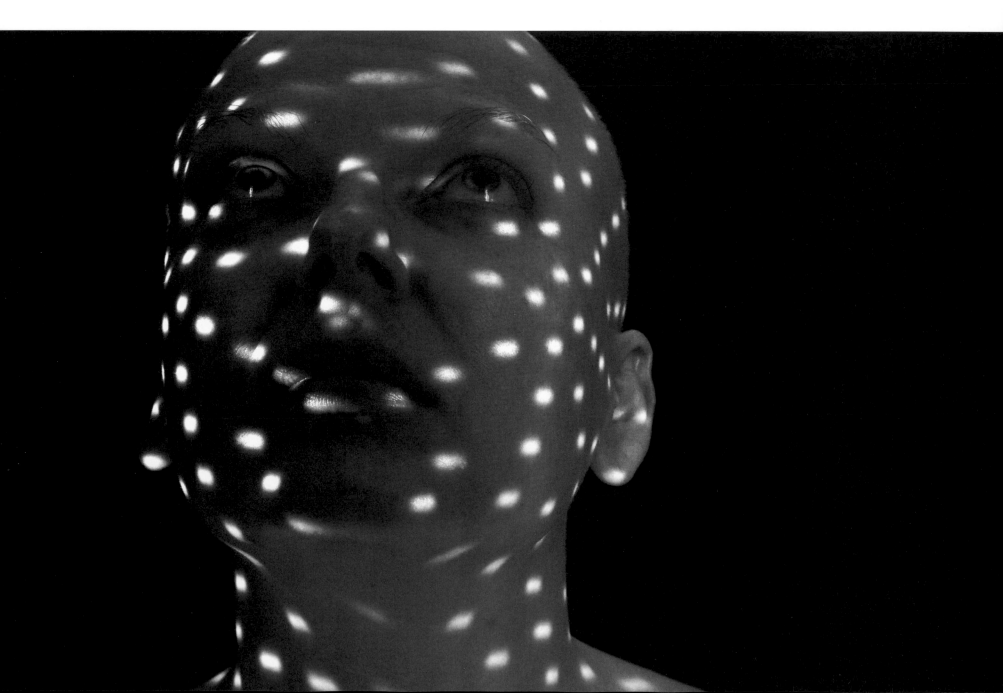

Over

Julie

Julie has Von Hippel-Lindau disease, a hereditary cancer-causing syndrome that results in her chronic renal cell carcinoma. Without huge medical advancements, her daughters face the same future.

Photographer
Kim Mallory
Abbortsford

Cindy

After undergoing a mastectomy for breast cancer in 2006, Cindy Bury likened herself to a unicorn, empowering herself to face the battle that was before her. Three years later another lump was found on the same side. Cindy has opted for natural healing and refuses to let the disease get the better of her.

Photographer
Arlene Simpson
Langley

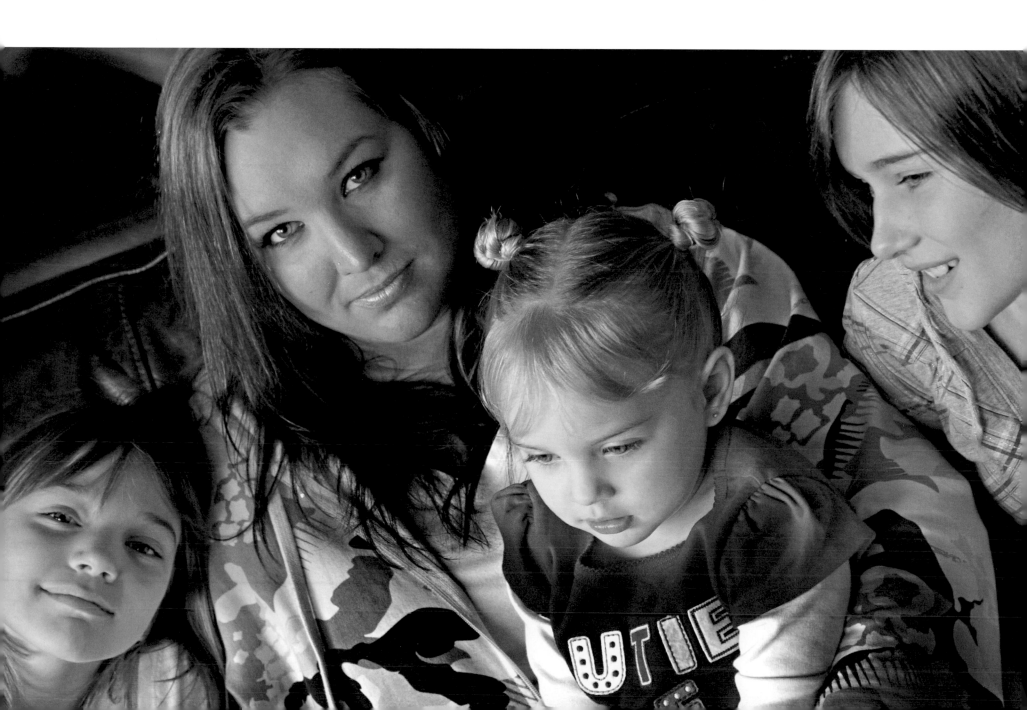

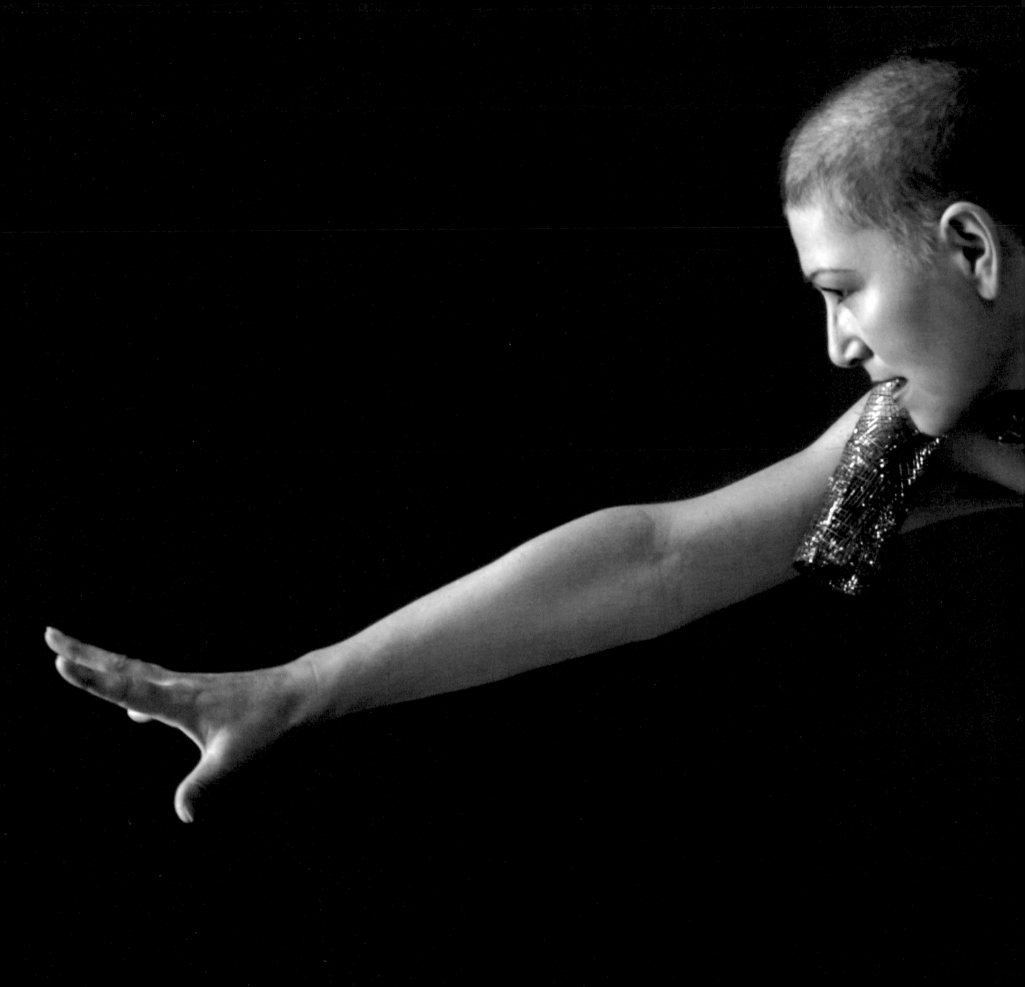

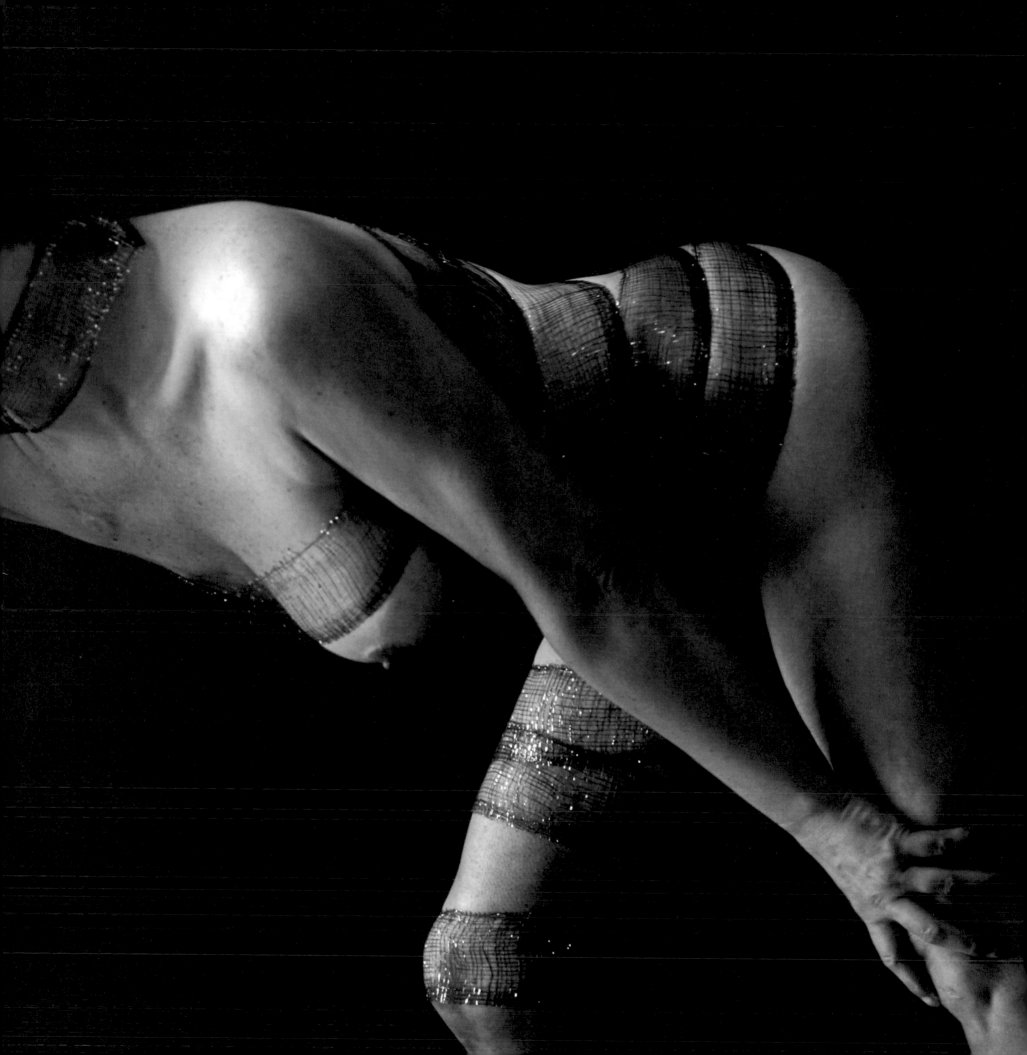

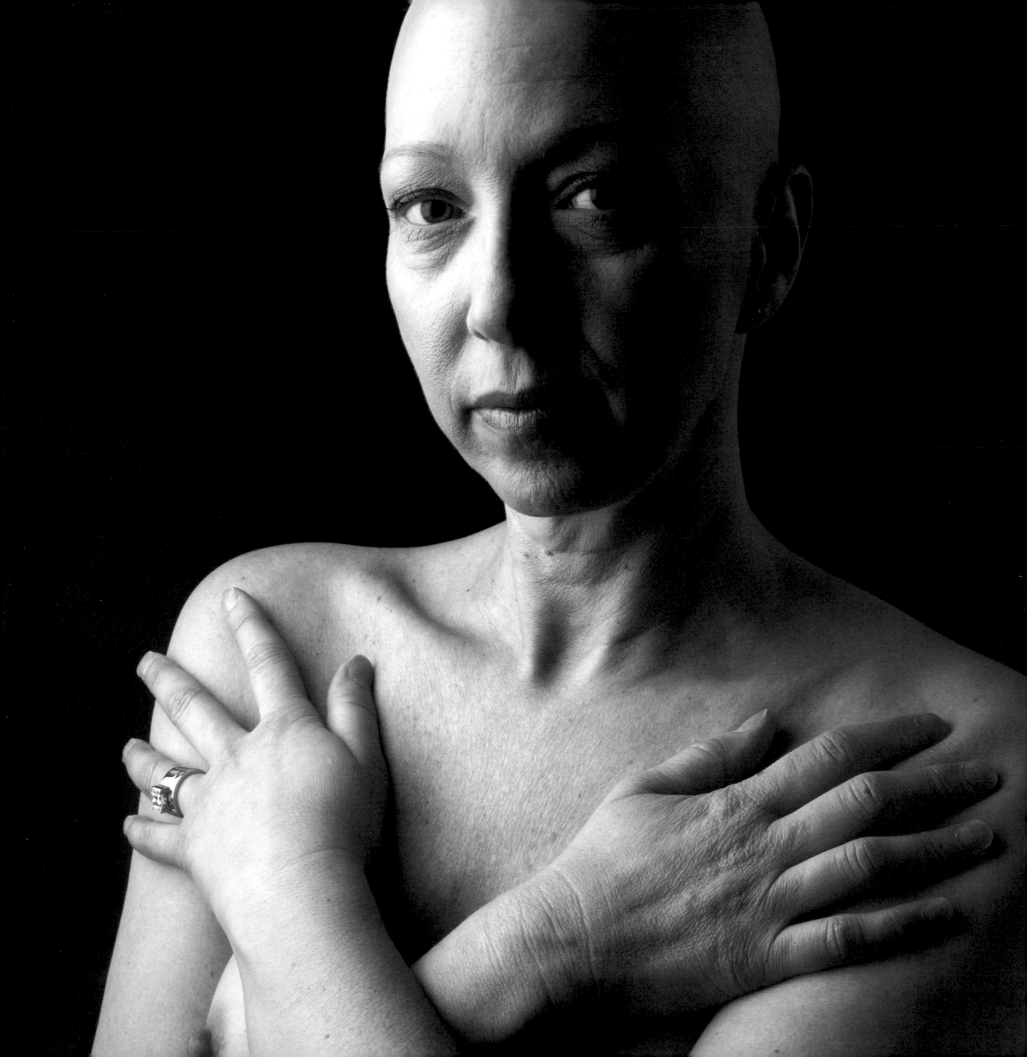

Opposite

Carolyn

Carolyn discovered she had breast cancer after tests for a bleeding nipple. Following a lumpectomy and auxiliary node dissection, she underwent chemotherapy, finishing March 2, 2010. Carolyn says, "The goal was just to get to the end of the chemo—now that I'm there and I start to feel better, as I look ahead, the lingering question is, will I survive this?"

Photographer
Wendy D
Vancouver

Madeleine

Ten years ago, while Madeleine De Little was battling breast cancer, her friend, artist Suzanne Northcott, offered to chronicle her cancer journey. Now a 10-year survivor, Madeleine is undergoing breast reconstruction. She says, "Now I understand that we never lose our beauty. It just becomes transformed."

Photographer
Michael Courtney
Fort Langley

Leah

Leah has survived breast cancer twice; she battled cancer while pregnant and recovered from open-heart surgery. She considers herself not merely a survivor, but a thriver, like so many of the courageous women she has met on her journey. Leah is a founding member of the Young and the Breastless group and volunteers for the Canadian Breast Cancer Foundation.

Photographer
Kimberly Mara
Vancouver

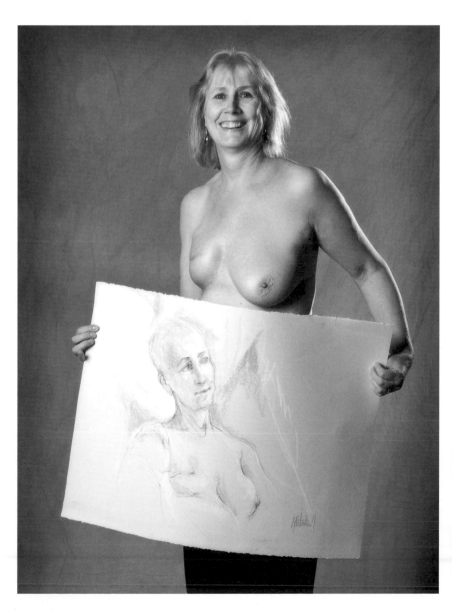

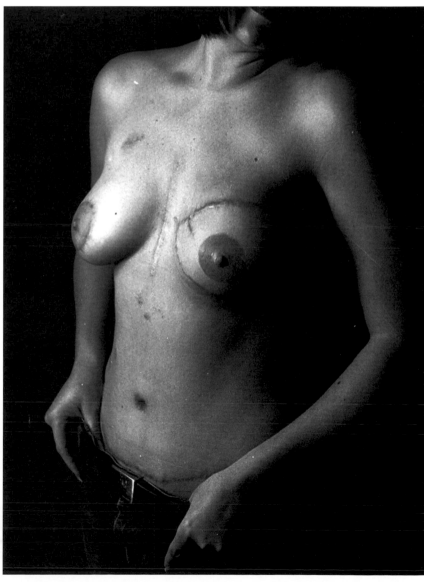

Leanne

Leanne Coombes cherishes
every moment she spends
with her two children, aged
four and six, after beating
breast cancer in 2007.

Photographer
Kyle Gehmlich
Chilliwack

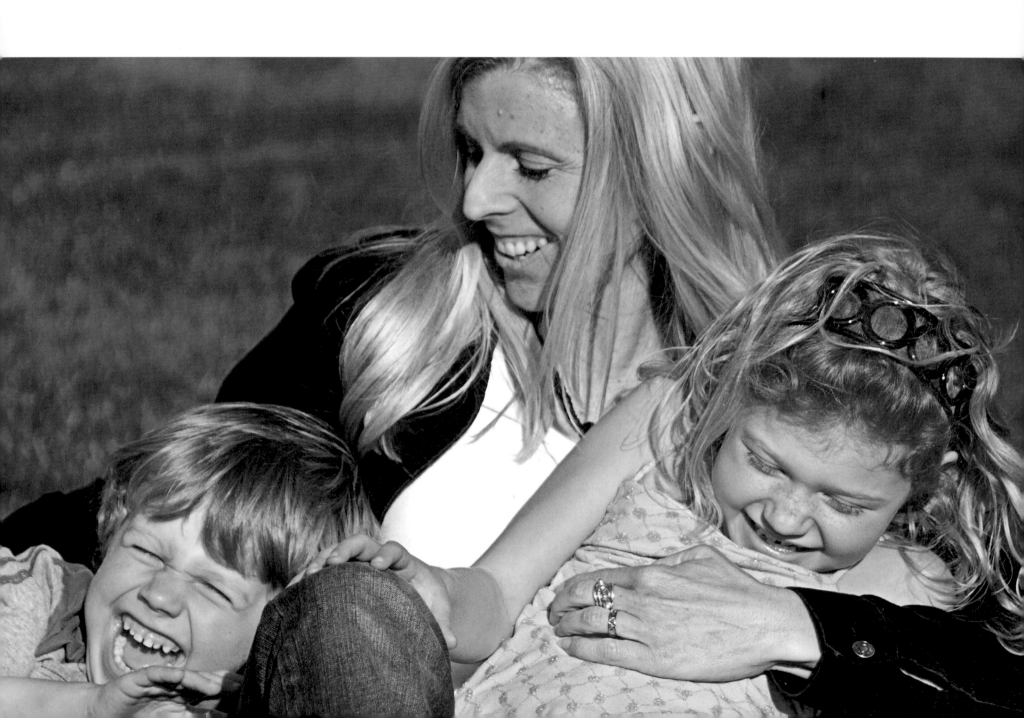

"Now that I start to feel better, as I look ahead,

the lingering question is, will I survive this?"

Carolyn Aronson

Lynda

Women from Lynda Paine's family after spending several hours working on her hair and makeup for the funeral. The five women were glad to have been part of what they found to be a freeing, powerful experience. Lynda had been diagnosed with colon cancer only one year earlier.

Photographer
Rick Collins
Chilliwack

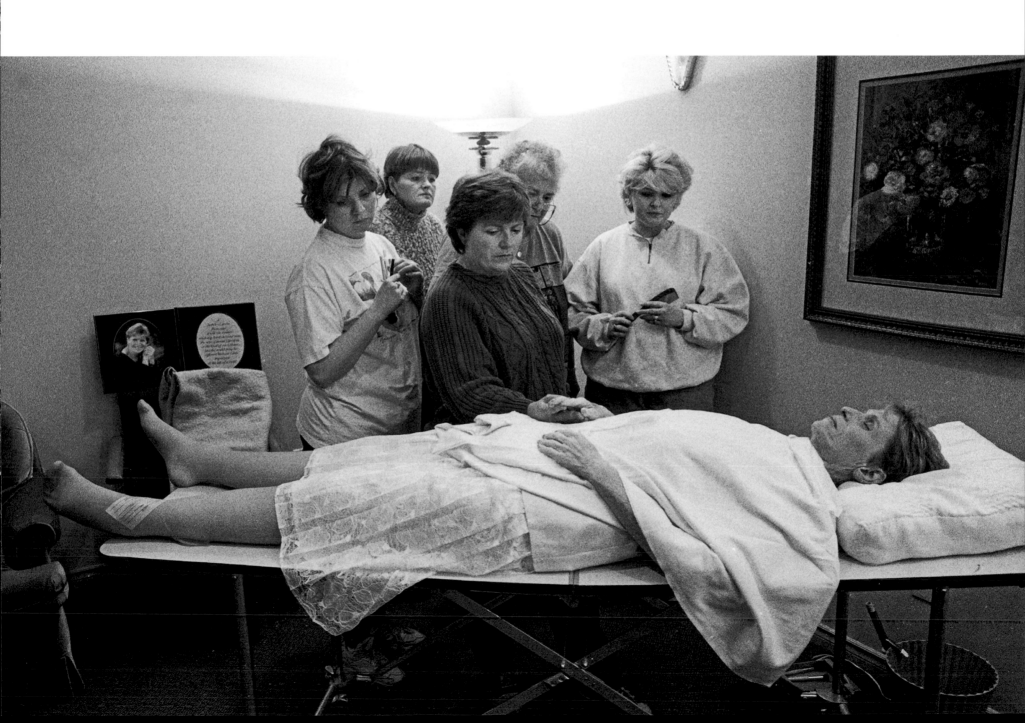

Row 1: Alfonso Arnold, Vancouver; Andrew Simpson, Langley; Andy Clark (3–5), Vancouver; Arlene Bishop, Comox; Barbara Belyea, Courtenay; Bryan Adams, Vancouver

Row 2: Daniel Sikorskyi (1–6), Victoria; Denise Everett (7–8), West Kelowna

Row 3: Doug Williams, Vancouver; Elaine Miller, Vancouver; Elizabeth Wong, Vancouver; Guy Warrington (4–6), Burnaby; Jenna Hauck (7–8), Chilliwack

Row 4: Jenna Hauck, Chilliwack; Jenny Garrett, Surrey; Jess Sloss, Vancouver; Jessica Offer, Kamloops; Julia Bowers, Kelowna; Karen McKinnon, Courtenay; Laura Leyshon (7–8), White Rock

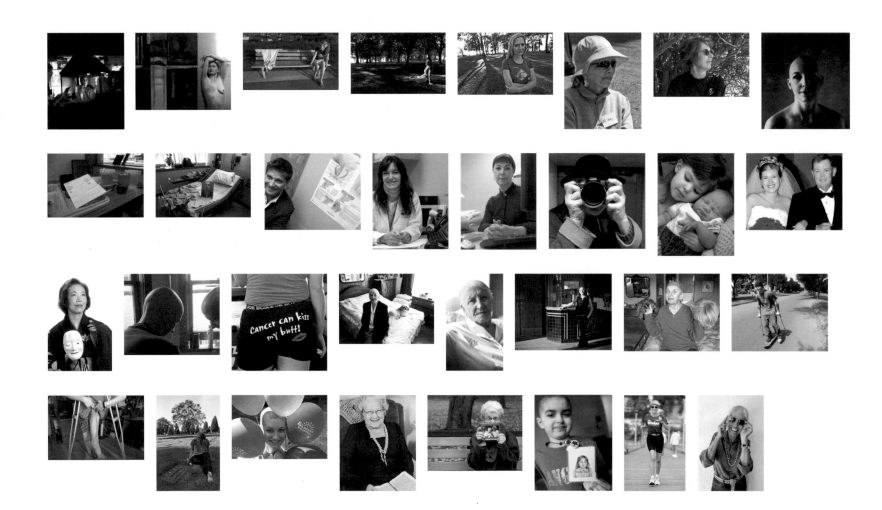

Row 1: Lauren Hammersley (1–4), Vancouver; Lucille Schubert, Vernon; Marie Seibel, Salmon Arm; Michael Courtney (7–8), Langley

Row 2: Michelle Morel, Prince George; Mikul Culver, Vancouver; Patrick Sullivan (3–4),Vancouver; Pierre Le Provost, Delta; Quinton Gordon, Cache Creek; Rafal Gerszak, Vancouver; Raymond Lum, Vancouver

Row 3: Sari McNamee, Langley; Spider Robinson, Bowen Island; Stacey Kushniruk, Vancouver; Teann Ingram, Prince George; Tesh Teshima, Vancouver; Travis F. Smith, Vancouver; Trevor Batstone, Maple Ridge; Trinity Berryman, Vancouver

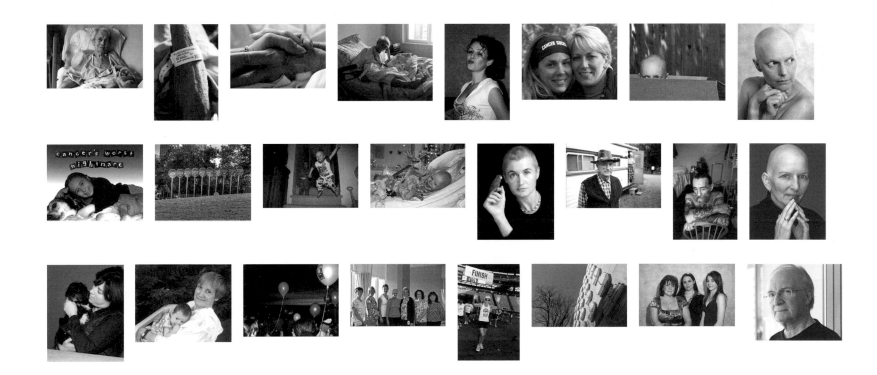

The Prairies

Alberta, Saskatchewan, and Manitoba

"I've been here before, I'm going to fight this. I am determined not to let this disease think it's winning."

Dionne Warner

Photographer
David Jay
Edmonton, Alberta

Sylvia

I Don't Have Time for This: Not only is this how Sylvia Soo felt while battling breast cancer but it's also the title of a documentary following five young breast cancer survivors as they go through treatment. Sylvia is one of those women.

Sylvia was just 25 when she was diagnosed with cancer, having returned from working in Korea to have a lump checked out. A biopsy revealed that she had stage 2 breast cancer.

"My initial thought was, 'Will I lose my hair?'" recalls Sylvia. "I had really long hair and the thought of losing it made me break down. I also had to deal with my mortality at just 25. I was a really busy person, I had so much on the go, so having that taken away from me was really hard."

The cancer had spread to two lymph nodes, which prompted the surgeon to present Sylvia with a difficult decision. She could opt for either a lumpectomy or a full mastectomy. A lumpectomy was less invasive, but there was a chance that it would not reveal the margins around the tumour and further surgery might be required.

"It was hard being given that choice. I had less than a week to think about it, so I was googling stuff and asking friends and then, the day before surgery, I decided to go with the mastectomy—and I'm glad I did. Six months later I started with reconstruction."

Six rounds of chemotherapy followed the surgery, which caused neuropathy in Sylvia's fingers and toes and caused her legs to swell up horribly. But it didn't stop Sylvia from keeping busy. She made a short film, *Dear Sister*, which was one of eight finalists at Toronto's 2009 Breast Film Festival; acted in the independent feature film *The Corrupted* (while undergoing chemotherapy); took part in The Scar Project, a breast cancer photo exhibition by New York fashion photographer David Jay; and captured footage of herself for *I Don't Have Time for This*.

After being given the all-clear from her doctors, Sylvia began writing a memoir/resource book with the working title *Cancer Fabulous*. Her vision of the book as an edgy, go-to resource for future survivors, patients, and the general public has involved interviewing dozens of young breast cancer survivors.

"When I was diagnosed with cancer, I couldn't find anything to prepare me for what was going to happen," says Sylvia. "This book will cover everything that young women can expect to go through, from coming to terms with the diagnosis to how it can affect relationships. It will be an uplifting book, with amazing stories."

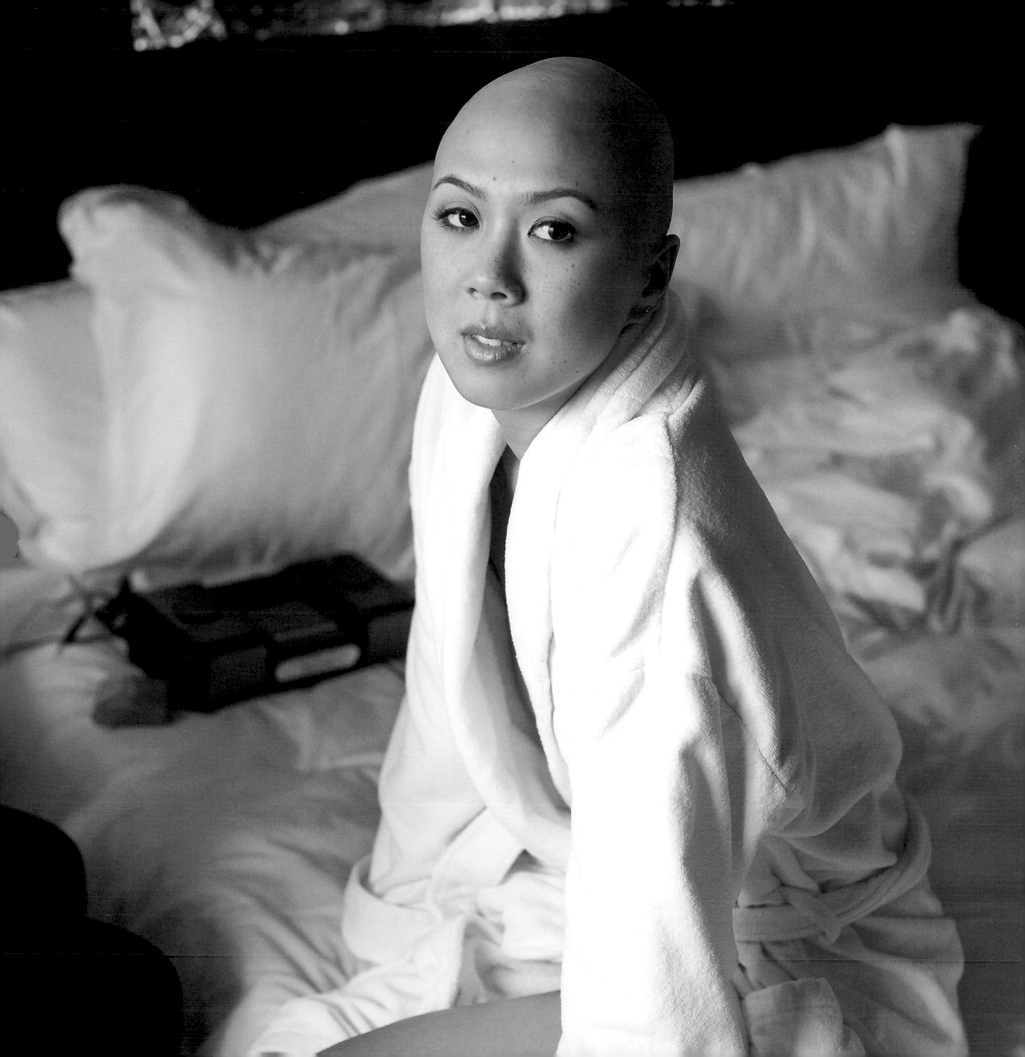

Lisa

Teresa Nuthall and her son Grayson are frozen in grief as they honour Teresa's sister, Lisa Murray, at the Canadian Cancer Society's Relay for Life in June 2007. Two months earlier, Lisa died of a rare form of cancer that attacked her connective tissue.

Photographer
Olivia Kachman
Wanham, Alberta

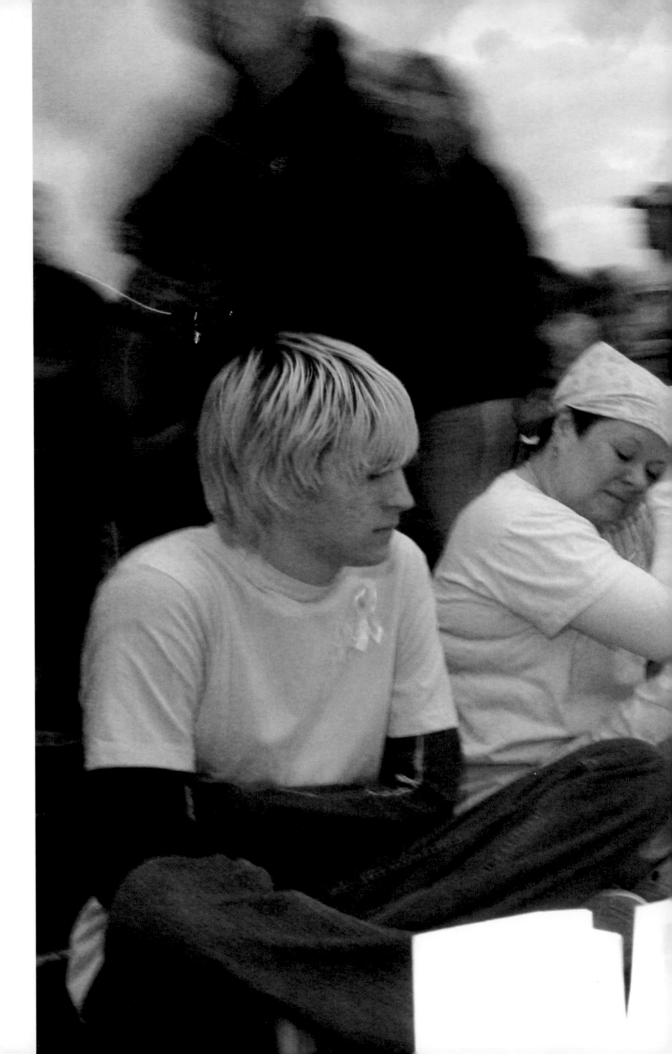

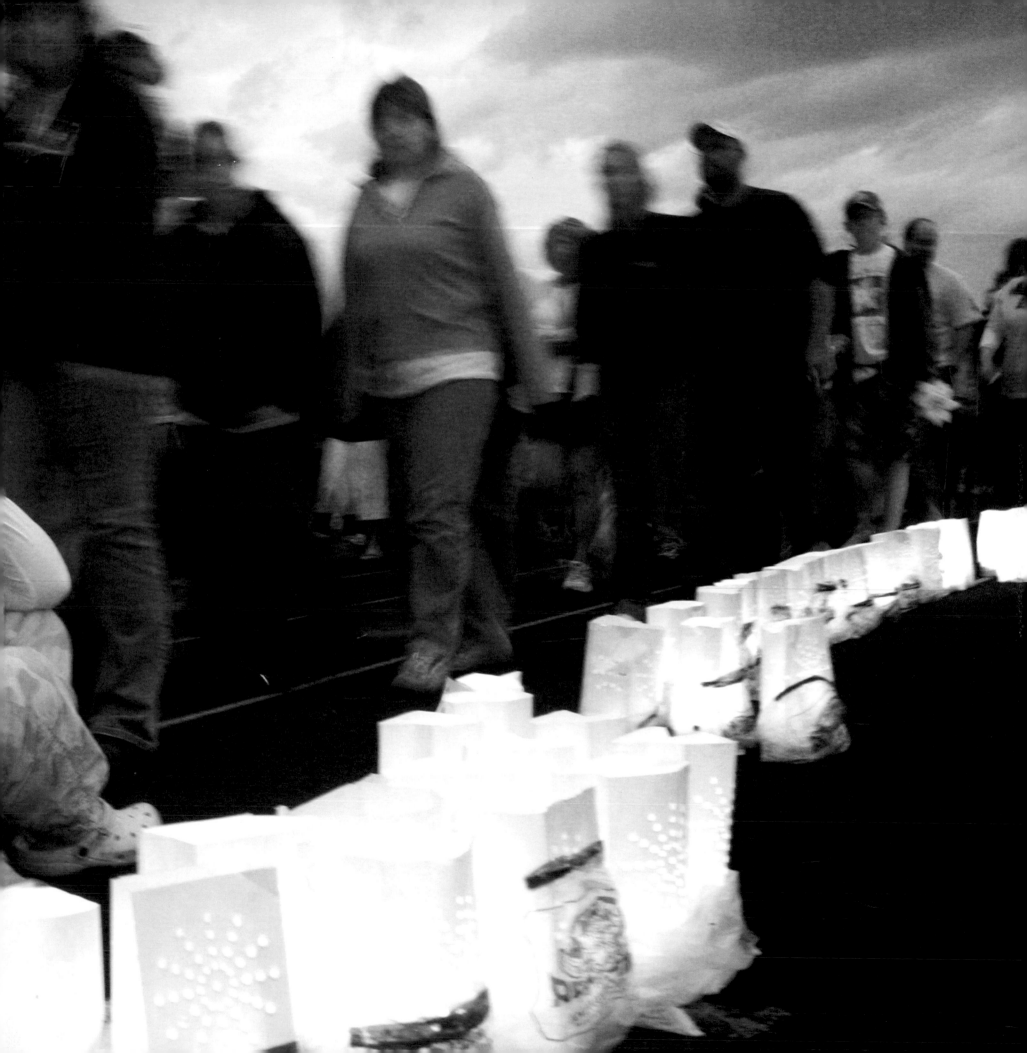

Photographer
Irene Tillusz
Regina, Saskatchewan

Dionne

When photographer Irene Tillusz submitted this photo of Dionne Warner with her husband, Graham, to *Cancer Connections* in 2007, Dionne's oncologist was already referring to her as a "walking miracle."

Dionne was a four-time cancer survivor, having successfully battled cancers of the breast (1995), brain (1997), and liver (twice, in 2001 and 2002). Chemotherapy and radiation had helped her to beat all four cancers and she regularly volunteered at a local cancer centre and attended a variety of cancer-related fundraisers.

By spring 2009, when *Cancer Connections* opened in her hometown of Regina, Dionne had been cancer-free for seven years. However, the shadow of cancer still loomed over her: "Every time I go for a checkup I get nervous. But I feel good, people say I look good, so I feel like I'm doing pretty well."

Six months later, after a routine checkup, Dionne got the news that she had hoped to never hear again: the cancer had returned. It was now in her back, pelvis, ribs, lung, and liver. And this time it was stage 4.

For many people, a first cancer diagnosis can be devastating, but to hear that you have cancer for the fifth time must be incredibly difficult to take. Not for Dionne: "I've been here before. I'm going to fight this."

With support from her husband Graham, Dionne became extremely proactive in her treatment. Doctors gave her a combination of drugs and chemotherapy; she also went to Mexico for a hyperthermia treatment where some of her blood was removed, heated, and then returned to the cancerous areas of her body. While there, she also radically changed her diet to low-fat as well as gluten- and sugar-free foods, and she began taking high doses of vitamin D daily.

Dionne decided to make her weekly chemotherapy session something to look forward to, instead of something to dread. "Graham and I dress up in a different theme each week. We've worn pink for breast cancer month and dressed as cowboys, flappers, and Olympians. We've had over 40 themes so far. The other patients love it. Graham takes lots of photos and then e-mails them in our weekly newsletter to all of our friends."

This positive attitude seems to be paying off. "The cancer is responding well," says Dionne. "I think it's been a combination of everything I've been doing. The tumours are starting to shrink and my back is feeling much better. I haven't felt the excruciating pain for a long time. I am determined not to let this disease think it's winning."

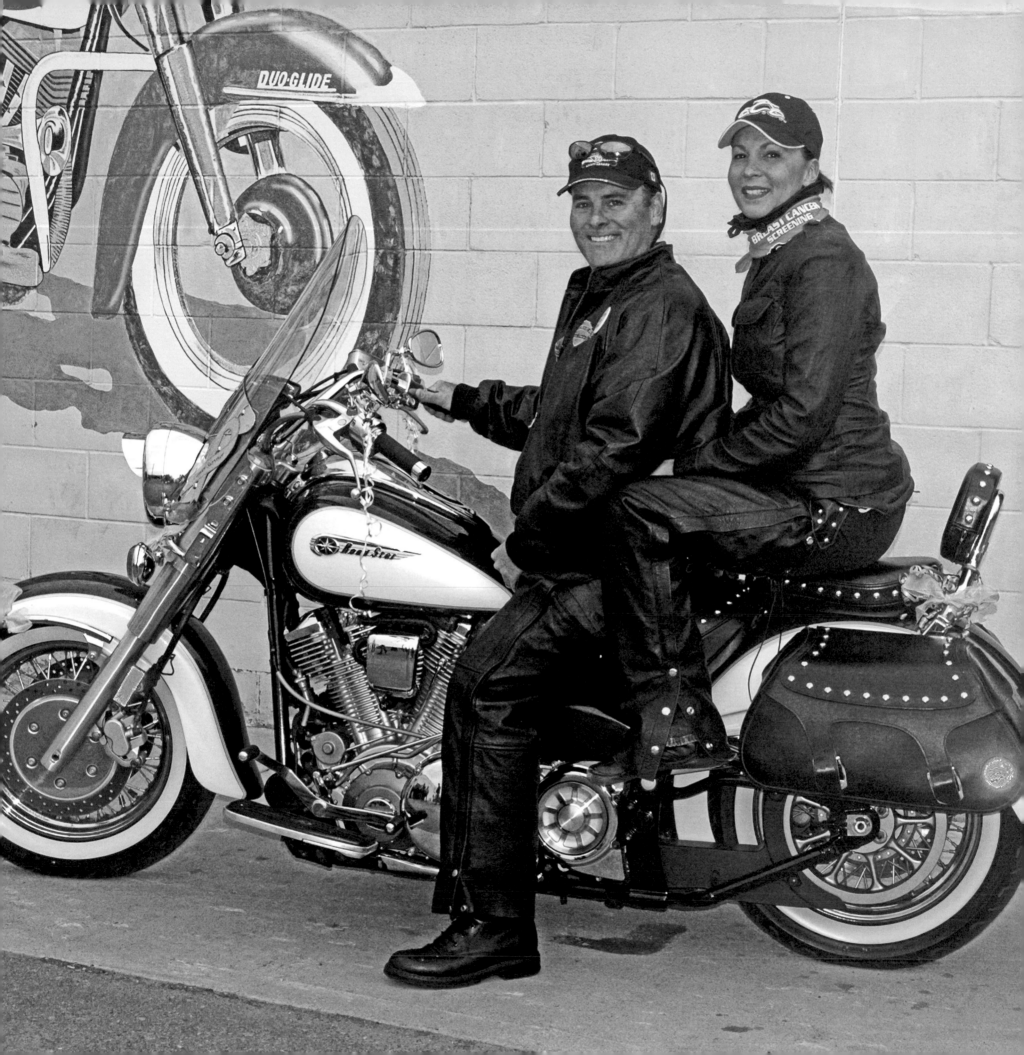

Angie and Ava

Angie Douville playing with her daughter Ava, three months after having a total hysterectomy for cervical cancer at age 31. Angie says, "Thanks to the birth of my daughter, the cancer was detected early and we both have each other. I want to thank all of the women before me and the research that helped me beat cervical cancer."

Photographer
Angie Douville
Regina, Saskatchewan

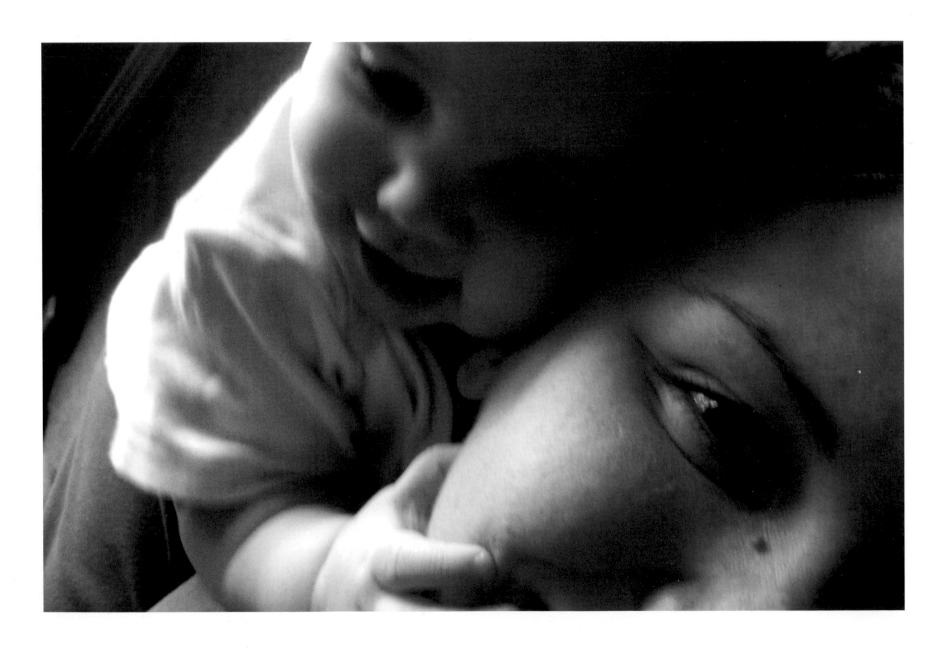

Kids Cancer Care Foundation

Photographer Matthew Cudmore was asked to take some photos at the Kids Cancer Care Foundation of Alberta summer camps. Children living with cancer attend the camps for free. "The Foundation does its best to help these kids just be kids," says Matthew. "It has a lasting effect on these children."

Photographer
Matthew Cudmore
Calgary, Alberta

Over left

Susan

Susan was diagnosed with advanced cervical cancer in 2007, in spite of having regular pap tests. She says, "My cancer was an invisible predator and treatment left invisible damage. How does one talk about that?"

Photographer
Andrew Sikorsky
Winnipeg, Manitoba

Over right

Ginette and Gabriella

Ginette, a breast cancer survivor, nursing her daughter Gabriella. She says, "I am 31 and found a lump on my breast on Gabriella's birthday. In March, I celebrated a year of nursing with one breast."

Photographer
Jessie Kimmel
Calgary, Alberta

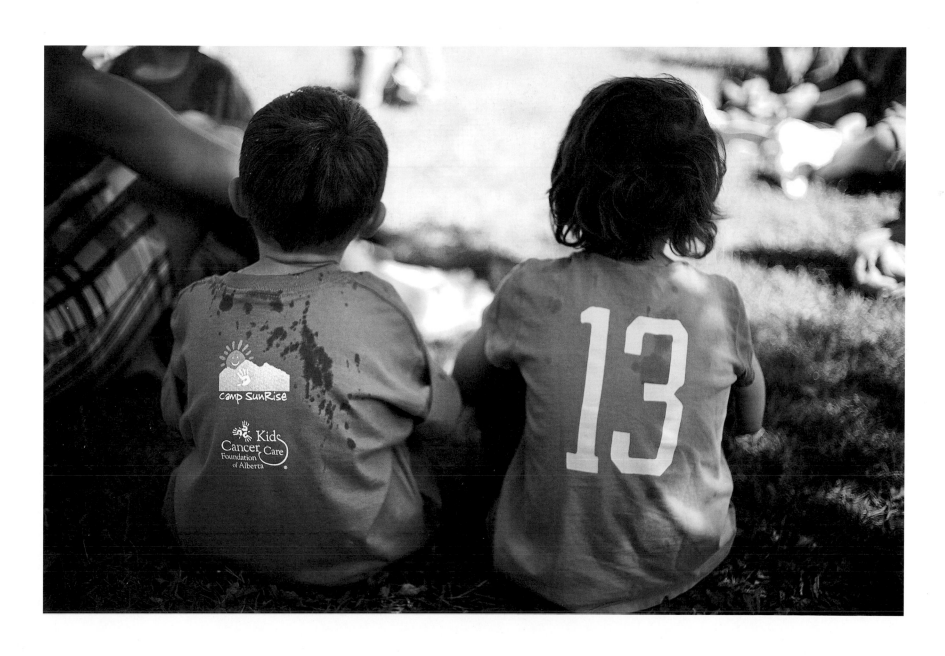

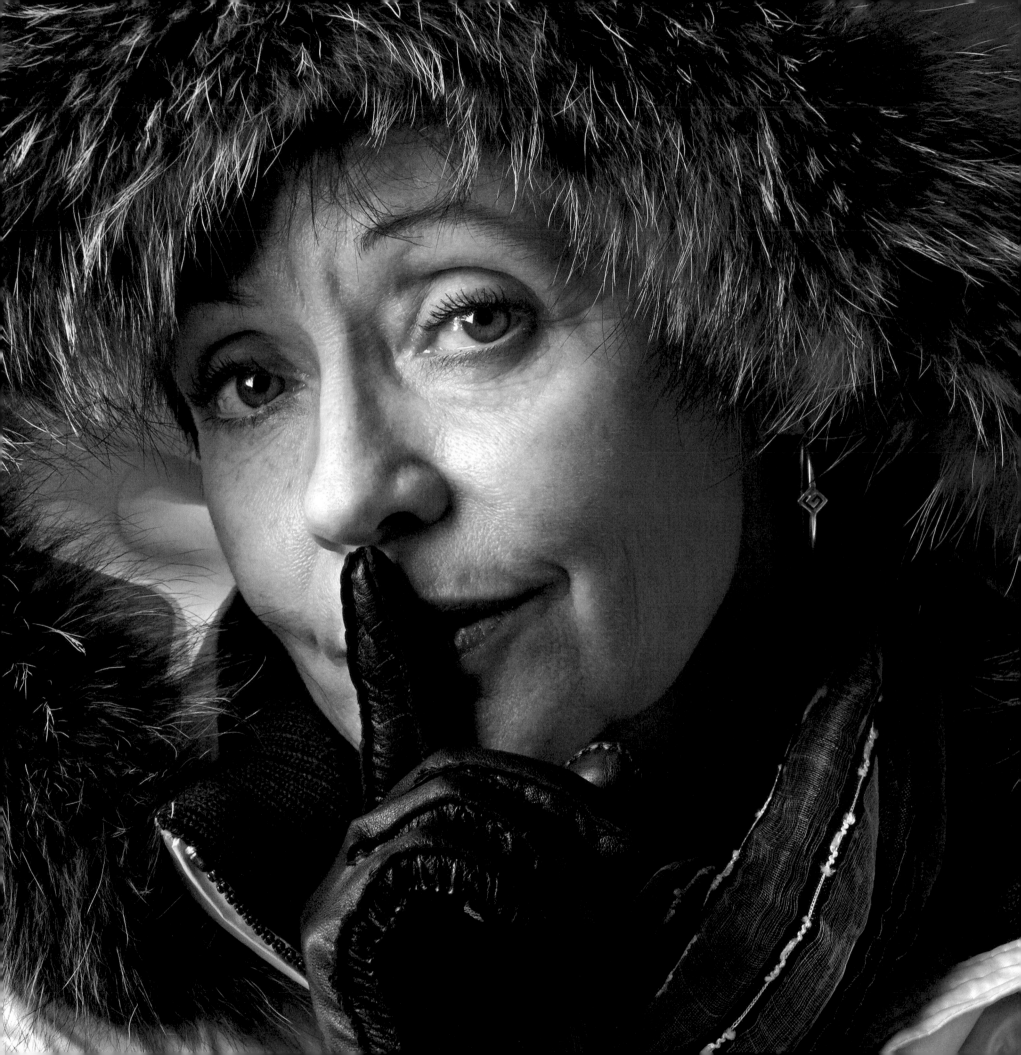

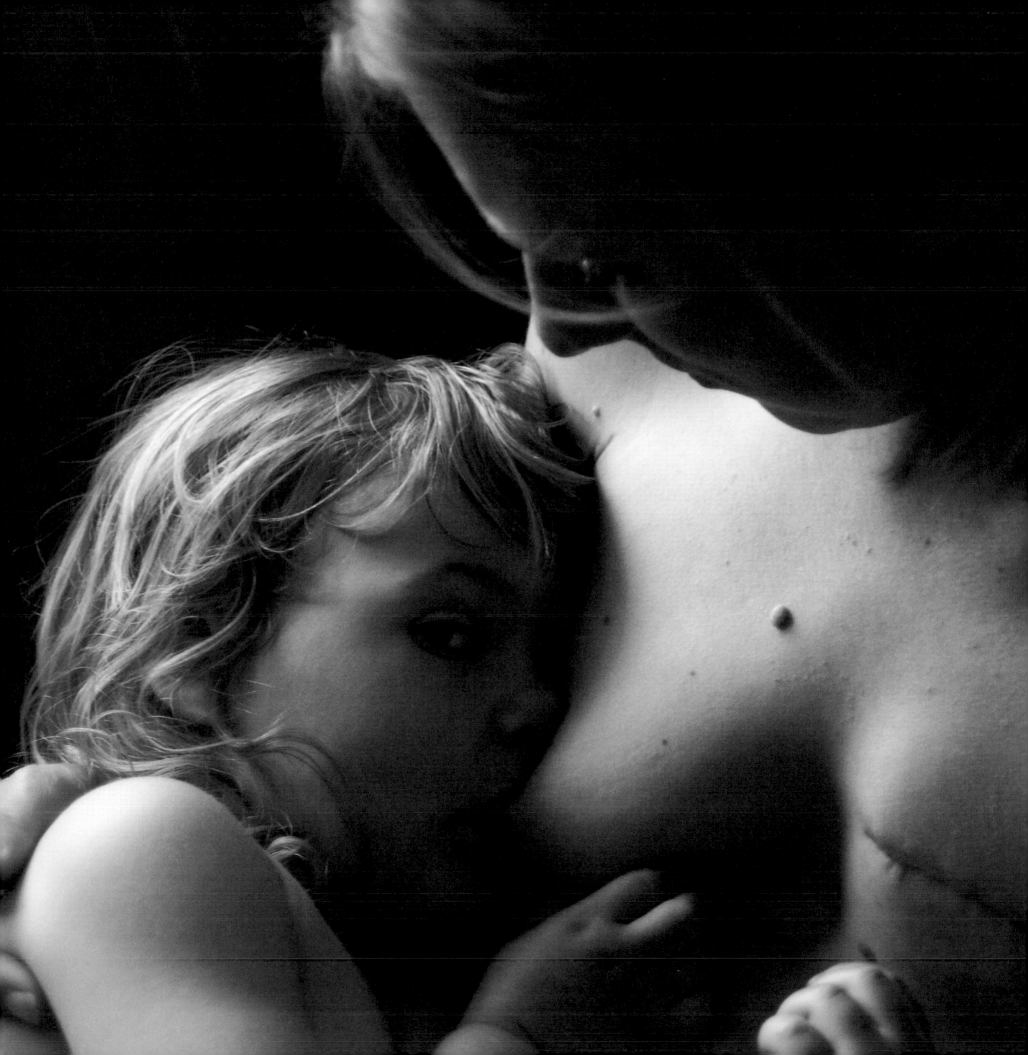

Jon

Jon Thordarson lost a kidney, a lung and one-third of his other lung to what started as treatable bladder cancer. The *Winnipeg Free Press* photo editor still rode 25 kilometres per day, six days a week. Sadly, Jon lost his eight-year battle in March 2010.

Photographer
Phil Hossack
Winnipeg, Manitoba

Wes and Jean

Wes Lysack, Calgary Stampeder and Grey Cup champion, fights cancer on behalf of his grandmother and number one fan, Jean Hillyard. Jean is a breast cancer survivor who wears her grandson's jersey along with a red Stetson and red cowboy boots to every game.

Photographer
Paul Austring
Calgary, Alberta

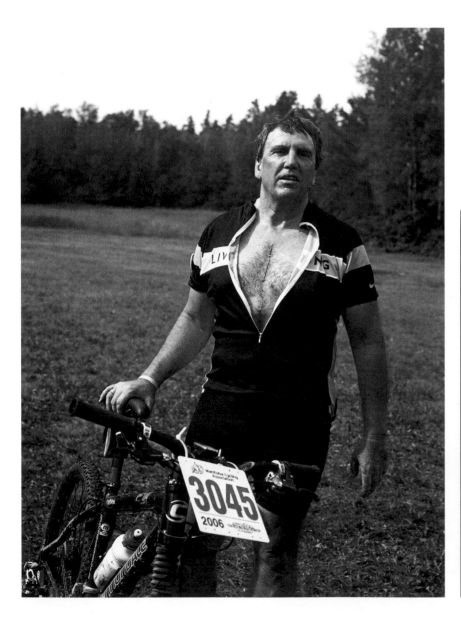

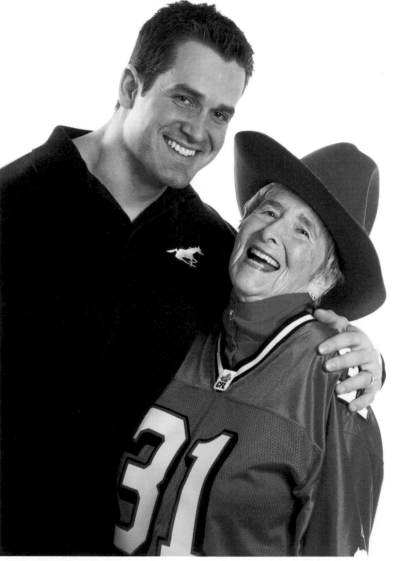

Braydon

Braydon Cushway, partici-
pating in his third Relay for
Life. Braydon was diagnosed
with clear cell sarcoma
of the kidney at the age of
10½ months. After opera-
tions that took out parts of
and whole internal organs,
extensive chemotherapy
and radiation, Braydon
is cancer-free. His parents
never gave up even
when the doctors said he
couldn't be cured.

Photographer
Heather Cushway
Moose Jaw, Saskatchewan

Sarah and Rachel

Sarah Denbigh with her
sister Rachel Chan, taken
on December 25, 2006.
Diagnosed at 30 with colon
cancer, Rachel was treated
with chemotherapy, but the
cancer was too aggressive.
Sarah asked their brother,
photographer Ian Jackson,
to take this photo moments
before Rachel died. "She
was my best friend,"
says Sarah.

Photographer
Ian Jackson
Edmonton, Alberta

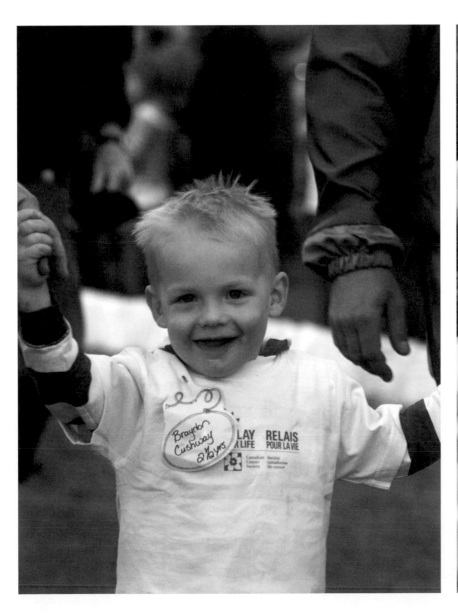

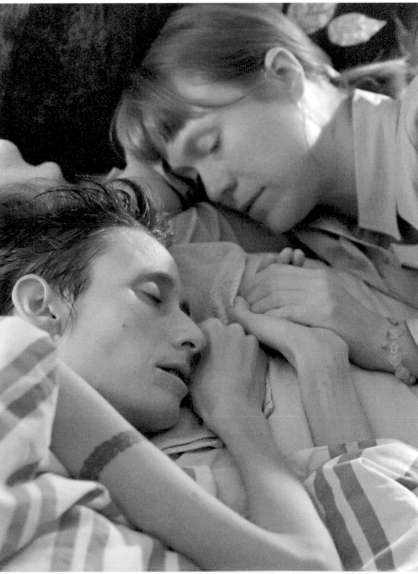

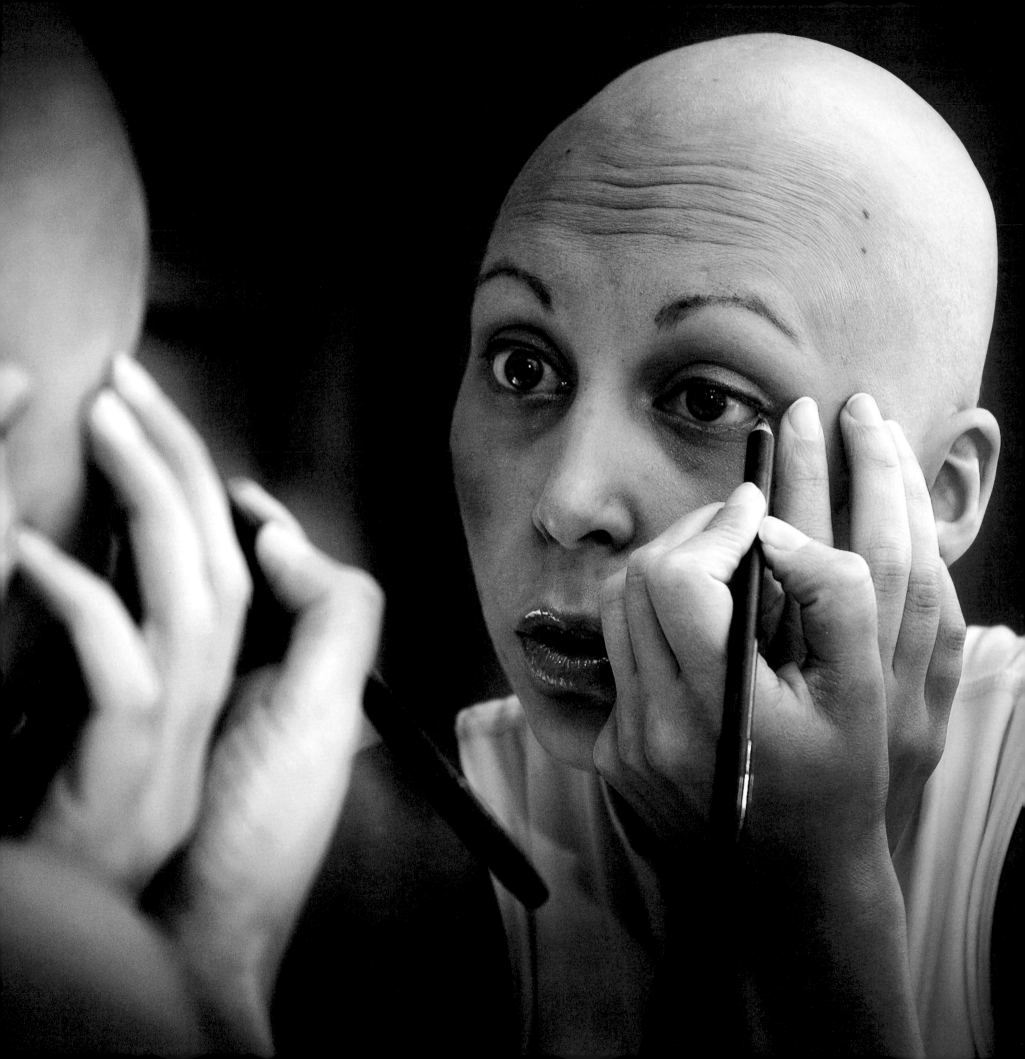

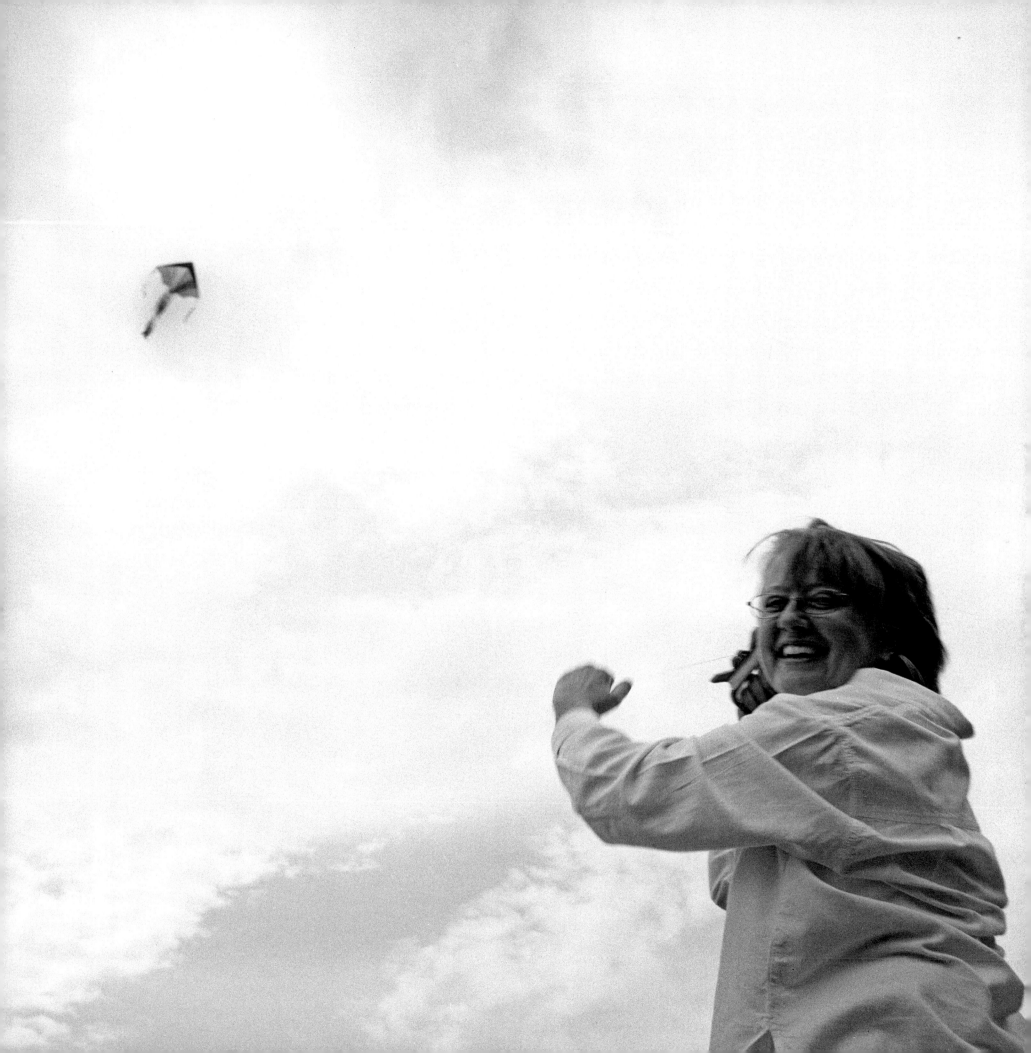

Previous left

Erin

Erin was diagnosed with breast cancer at 24. At 26, she was pronounced terminal but continued to explore alternative treatments, which dramatically improved her quality of life. Sadly, Erin passed away in June 2008.

Photographer
Aaron Vincent Elkaim
Winnipeg, Manitoba

Previous right

Noreen

Having undergone a mastectomy to treat her breast cancer, the disease returned in Noreen Gerbrandt's spine. Although it is treatable, it is not curable. Her lifelong dream was to fly a kite.

Photographer
Phil Hossack
Winnipeg, Manitoba

Josh

Josh Leslie learned to play the violin after his mother, Sue, died of cancer at the age of 29. He plays for her when he visits her gravesite.

Photographer
Colin Corneau
Minnedosa, Manitoba

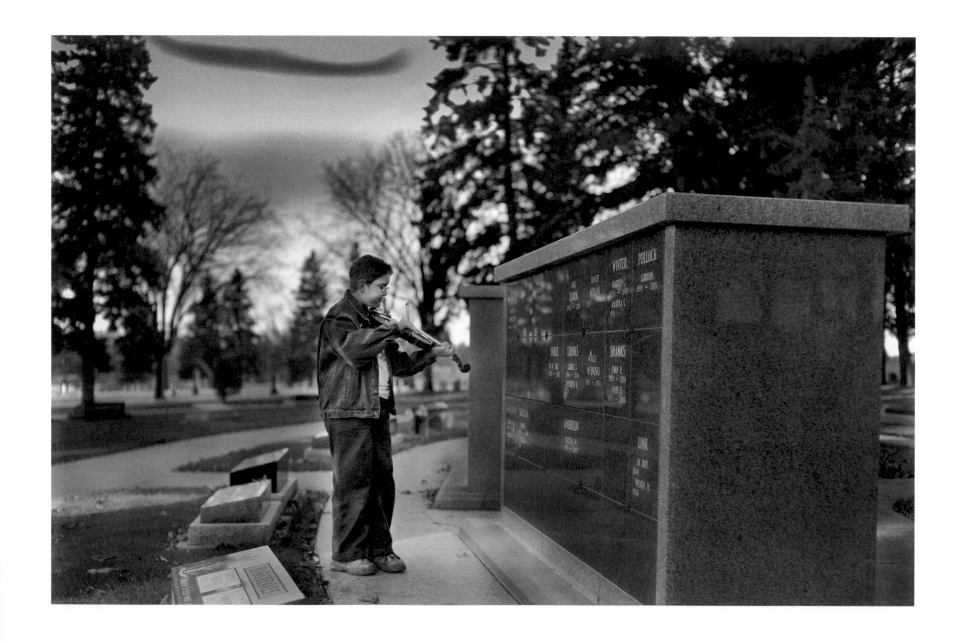

Matthew

Wearing number 4, Matthew Hower pursued his love of hockey cheered on by his mom Mary, dad Tim, and big sister Lauren. He continued to play for the Cardinals despite being treated for neuroblastoma. He was a huge Canadiens fan and family and friends honoured the eight-year-old's passion by wearing jerseys at his funeral.

Photographer
Andrew Sikorsky
Winnipeg, Manitoba

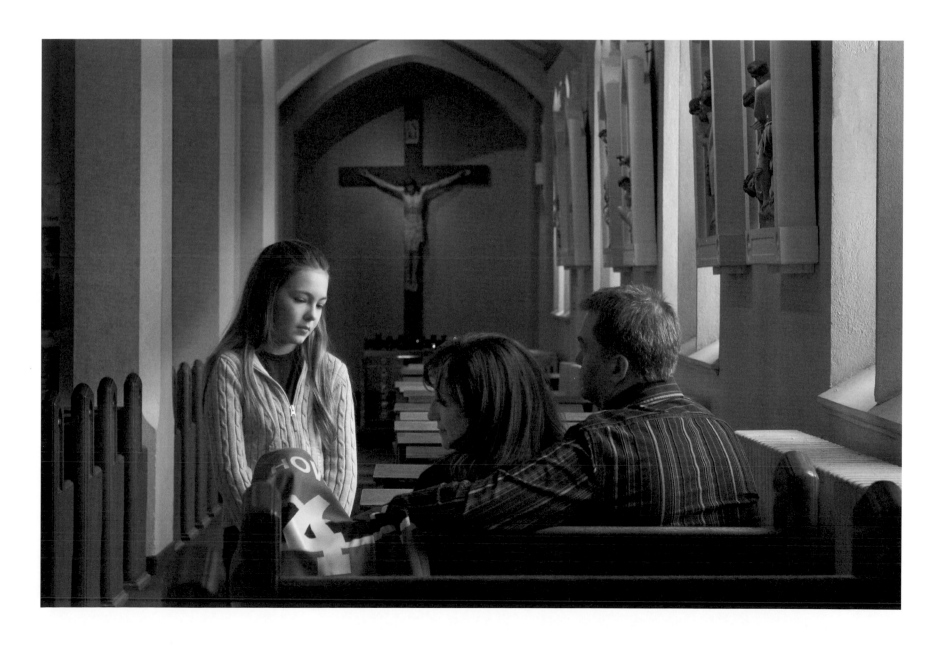

Opposite

Eli

Nine-year-old Eli at the dragon boat races. His mother is a breast cancer survivor and competes with the "Sistership Calgary" racing team.

Photographer
Rita Gore
Cochrane, Alberta

Jim

Jim, a pilot who flew with the Canadian Forces Snowbirds, with his beloved grandson AJ. In October 2007, Jim was told he had metastatic pancreatic cancer and was given three to six months to live. He defied the odds and lived until January 2, 2009. "We miss him dearly," says his wife, photographer Mary Ann.

Photographer
Mary Ann Fowler
Winnipeg, Manitoba

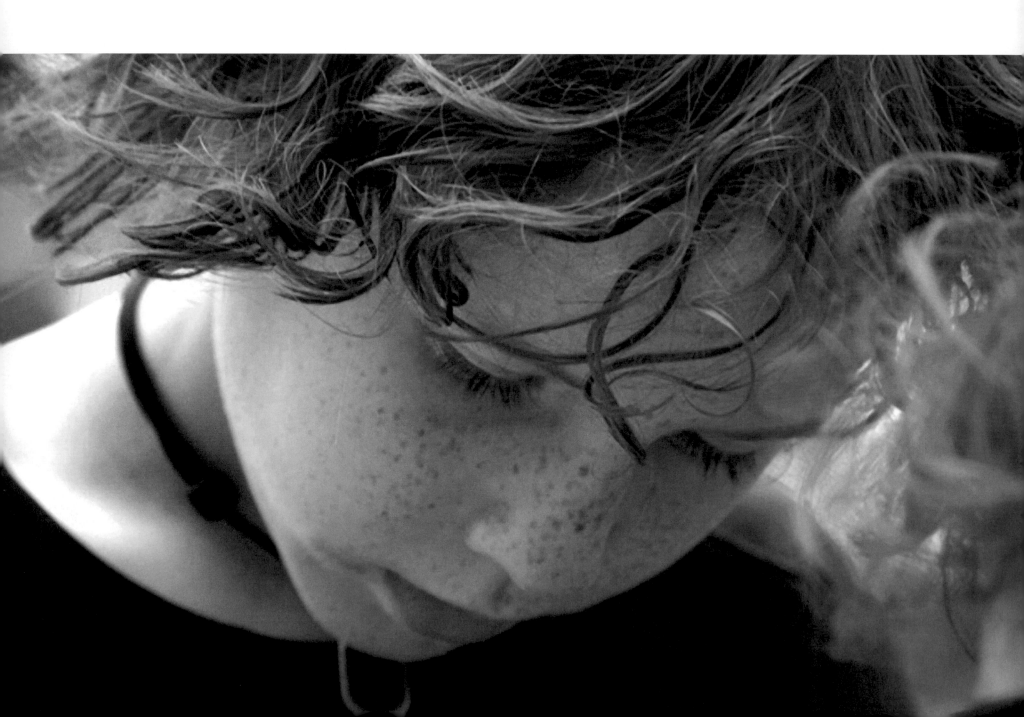

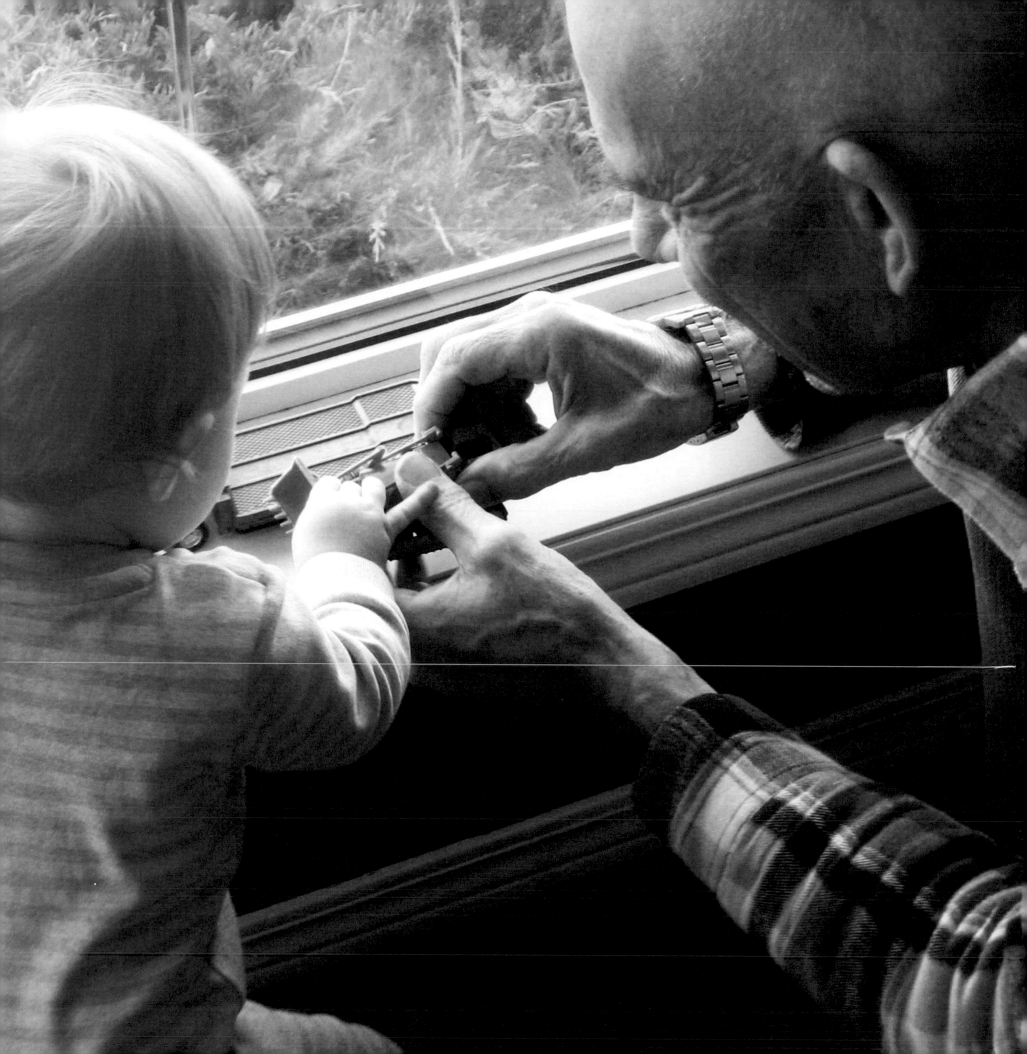

Row 1: Aaron Whitfield (1–2), Calgary, Alberta; Aaron Whitfield, Edmonton, Alberta; Andrew Querner, Canmore, Alberta; Anna Hunter, Edmonton, Alberta; Bert Luit, Winnipeg, Manitoba; Blayne Taylor (7–8), Calgary, Alberta

Row 2: Blayne Taylor, Calgary, Alberta; Bob Todrick, Edmonton, Alberta; Brenda Castonguay, Calgary, Alberta; Brian J. Gavriloff, (4–7), Edmonton, Alberta; Cal Fehr, Regina, Saskatchewan

Row 3: Carrie Carino, Winnipeg, Manitoba; Chad Mario, Regina, Saskatchewan; Colleen Hughes (3–4), Calgary, Alberta; Daniel Hayduk (5–6), Edmonton, Alberta; Darlene Gray, Regina, Saskatchewan; David Hou, Winnipeg, Manitoba

Row 4: David Hou; Winnipeg, Manitoba; Greg Fulmes, Calgary, Alberta; Holly Gray, Calgary, Alberta; Ian Jackson, Edmonton, Alberta; Ina Borger, Winnipeg, Manitoba; Jessica Korte, Humboldt, Saskatchewan; Jessie Kimmel, Calgary, Alberta; Judy Steinke, Wawota, Saskatchewan

Row 5: Justen Lacoursiere, Calgary, Alberta; Kirby Penner (2–5), Morden, Manitoba; Marianne Helm, Winnipeg, Manitoba; Mark Derry, Calgary, Alberta; Matea Tuhter, Winnipeg, Manitoba

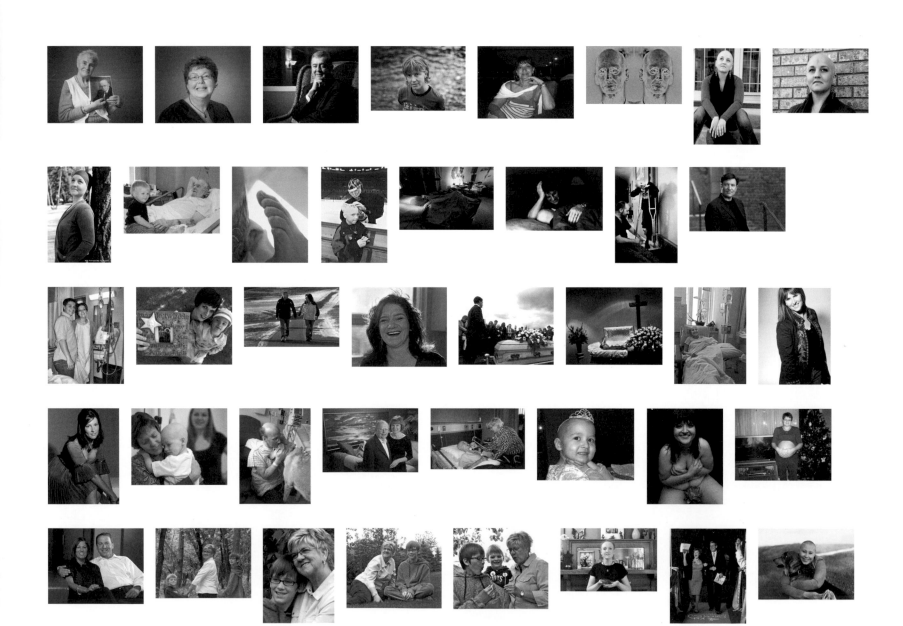

Row 1: Matthew Cudmore, Calgary, Alberta; Melanie Nargang, Regina, Saskatchewan; Merri-Lou Paterson, Winnipeg, Manitoba; Mirriam Staffen, Regina, Saskatchewan; Monique Westra, Veronica Wisniewska, Owen Melenka, Calgary, Alberta; Nancy Chambers, Drayton Valley, Alberta; Patricia Hancock, Yorkton, Saskatchewan; Paulette Kowalchuk, Winnipeg, Manitoba

Row 2: Pete Stepaniuk, Regina, Saskatchewan; Peter Ciechanowski, Edmonton, Alberta; Phil Hossack (3–4), Winnipeg, Manitoba; Rita Gore (5–7), Beaver Lodge, Alberta; Rita Gore, Calgary, Alberta

Row 3: Rita Gore, Calgary, Alberta; Ryan Holland, Calgary, Alberta; Serena Froese, Winnipeg, Manitoba; Sheryl Raymond, Regina, Saskatchewan; Tom Dykstra, Winnipeg, Manitoba; Tom Thomson, Winnipeg, Manitoba; Vance Lester, Saskatoon, Saskatchewan; Victor Jarman, Winnipeg, Manitoba

Row 4: Wanda Campbell (1–2), Regina, Saskatchewan

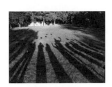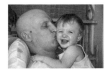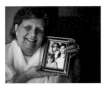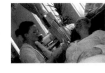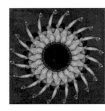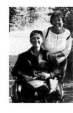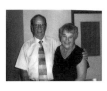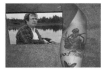
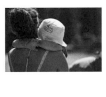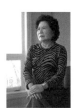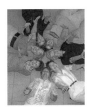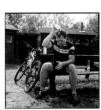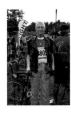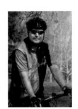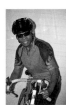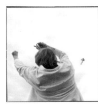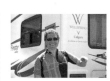
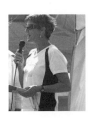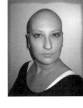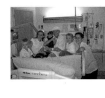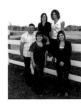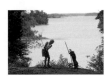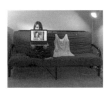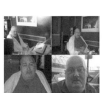
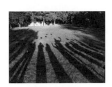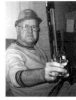

Ontario

"Life has changed, but there is still much joy."

Dave Jarrett

Photographer
Marilyn Jarrett
Oakville

Dave

This photo of Dave Jarrett and his granddaughter, Franca, taken by Dave's wife, Marilyn, was the image chosen for the information billboard that toured the country with the *Cancer Connections* exhibition. When Marilyn saw the poster at the launch of the show in Toronto, she was taken aback.

"I knew PhotoSensitive wanted to use the photo for some sort of promotion," she says, "but I will never forget walking across Nathan Phillips Square and my son Tynan pointing at this huge poster and saying, 'Mom, look!' I had no idea it was going to be so big."

The Jarretts were thrilled by their involvement with the exhibition. "I found it all to be a fabulous, exciting, and mind-boggling experience," says Marilyn. "Davey enjoyed it more because he was so proud of my photography and he loved to see how excited Franca was by the whole thing."

Dave's cancer journey had begun in January 2006, after quadruple bypass surgery following a heart attack. Shortly after the operation, Dave thought he had a cavity developing, but he wasn't allowed to have any dental work carried out until six months after the operation. As soon as possible, he visited a dentist, who immediately referred him to an oral surgeon. The biopsy revealed cancer of the jaw.

At the initial diagnosis, the cancer was stage 2–3; two months later, at the time of surgery, it had grown to stage 3–4. "The cancer was really aggressive," says Marilyn. "In that short time it went from a feeling of discomfort to his cheek puffing out."

During the 12-hour surgery, when the cancer and part of Dave's jaw were removed, muscle and skin from his shoulder were used to rebuild his jaw. Although the operation successfully removed the cancer, serious complications arose that brought on other illnesses over the next few years, leading to Dave passing away in January 2010.

"Davey was never one to complain," says Marilyn. "In those last years he always found much to enjoy, even though he had to give up so much. He continued working, right up to the end, and enjoyed talking with the kids and watching his grandchildren grow. He had a wonderful sense of humour and always had the gift of enjoying the moment. He was always more interested in the comfort of those around him than his own."

Franca has this photo on her bedroom wall and has placed origami stars around it. "She loves to look at it every day," says Marilyn, "and remember the good times they had together."

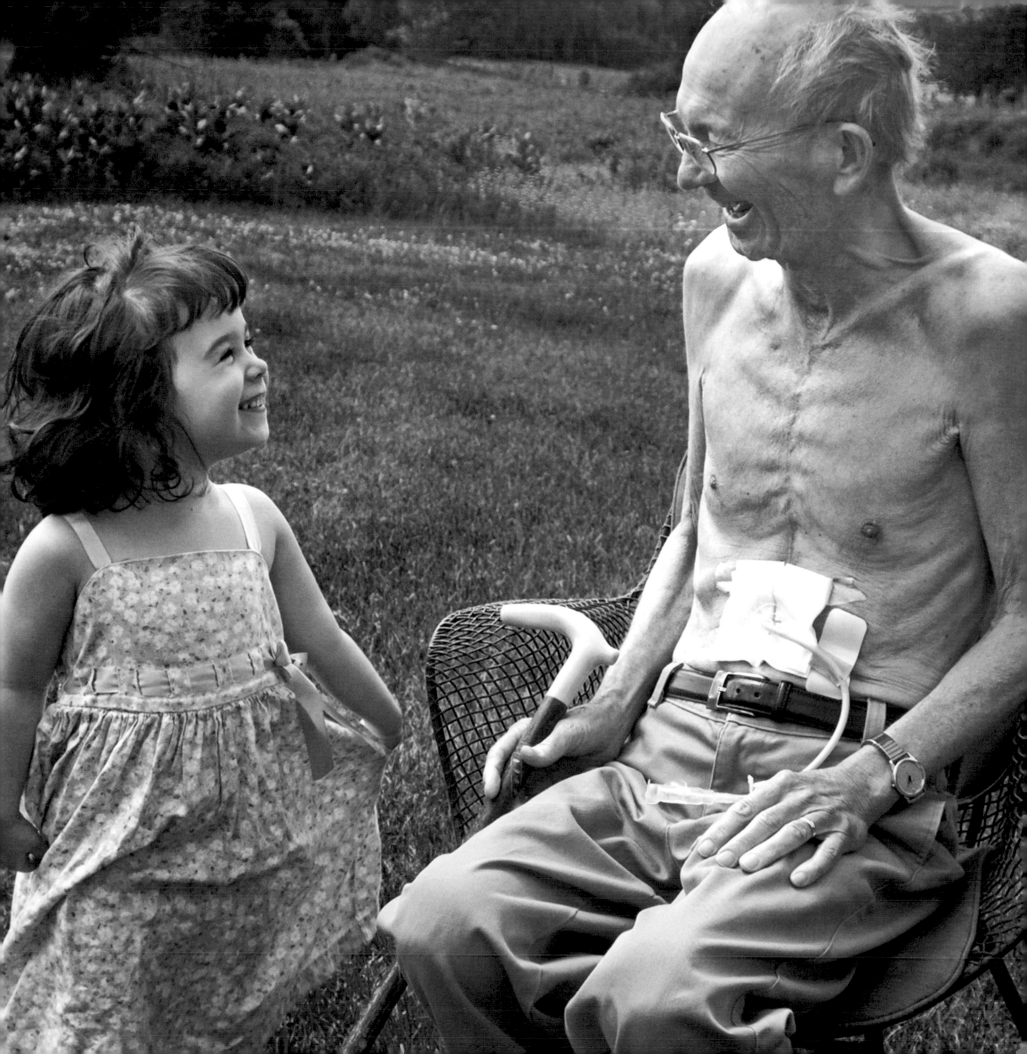

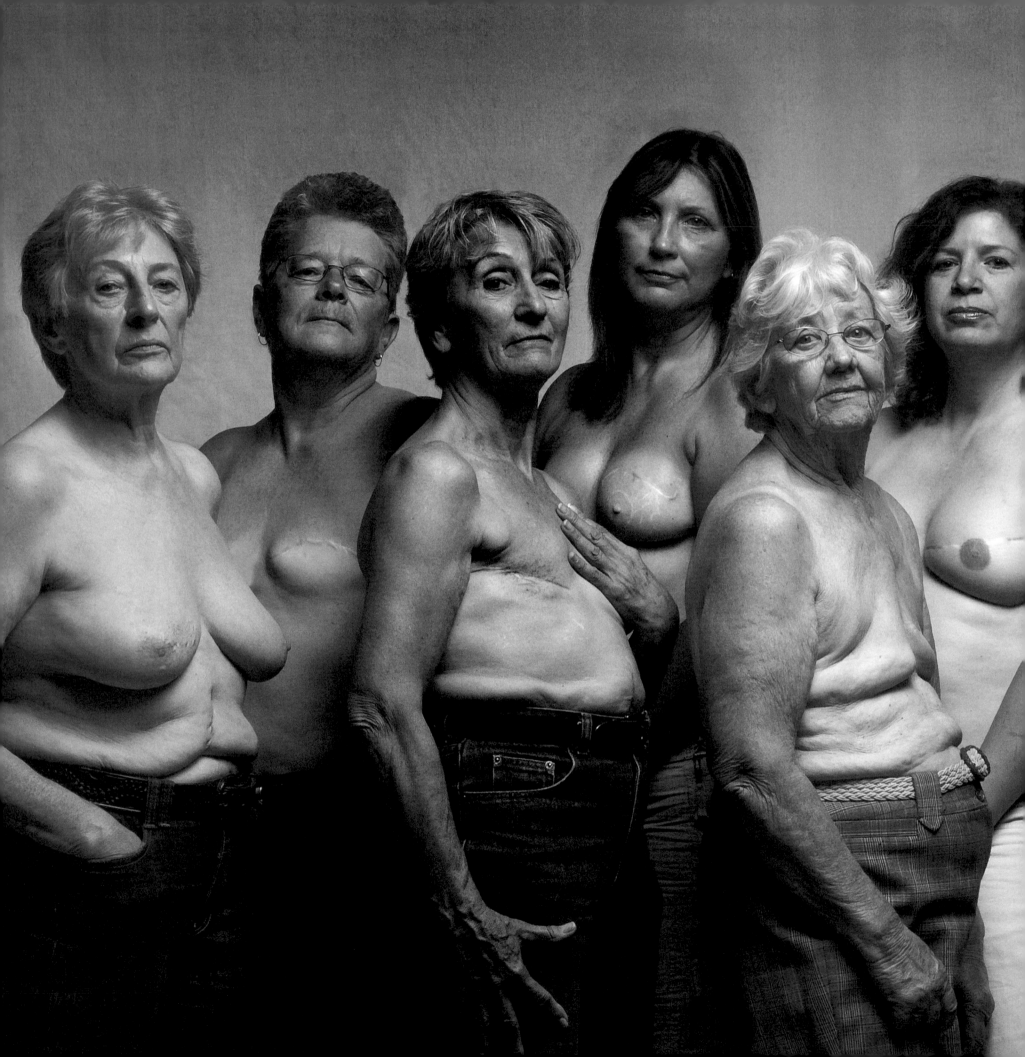

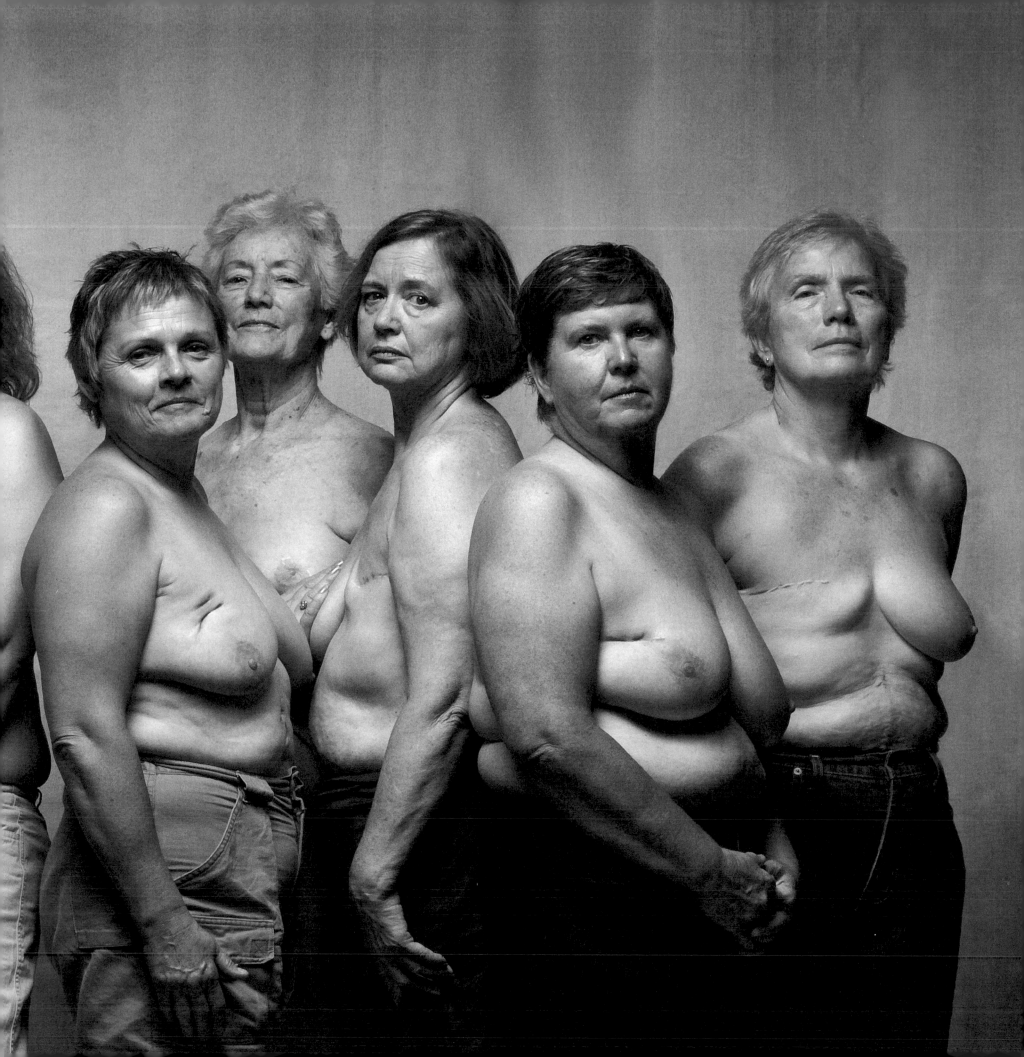

Previous

Survivor Thrivers

Eleven members of the
"Survivor Thrivers" dragon
boat team, a group
of women who are breast
cancer survivors.

Photographer
Gary Mulcahey
Port Hope

Loretta

Loretta, a breast cancer
survivor, with her
daughter Jenna. Loretta
was diagnosed in 2000, had
four months of chemotherapy
and radiation, and spent 10
months without hair. She has
now been cancer-free for
eight years.

Photographer
Cathy Chatterton
Douro

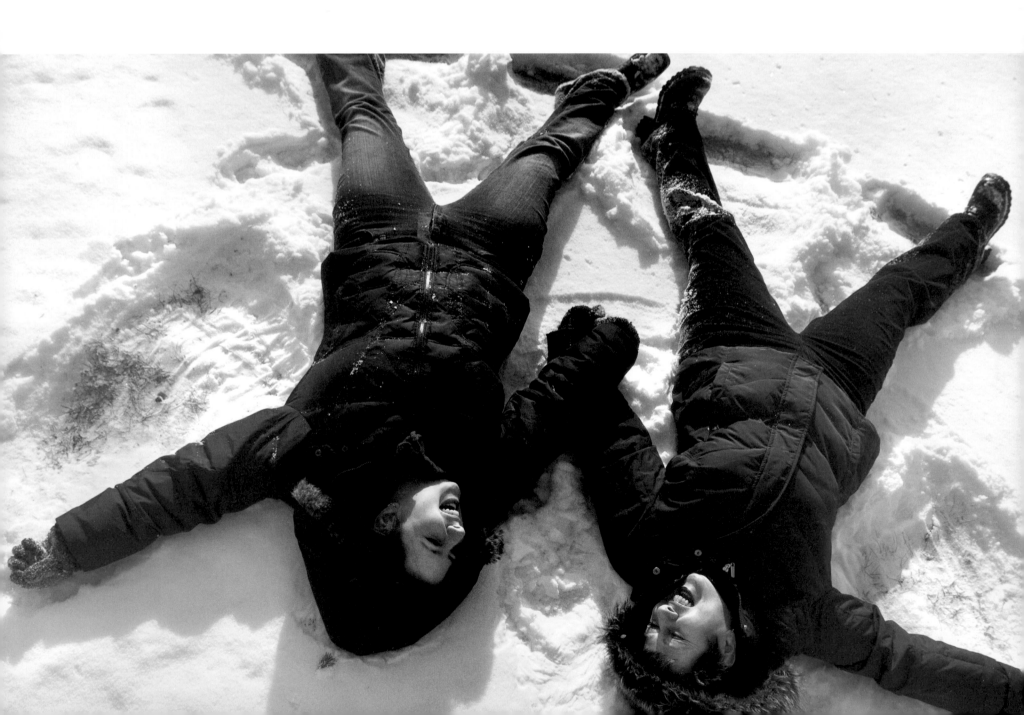

Elgin-Alexander

Two-year-old Elgin-Alexander,
seen here with his parents,
was diagnosed with neuroblastoma in January 2005.
Despite many attempts to
cure Elgin-Alexander of the
disease, he succumbed
to his illness in May 2007.

Photographer
Ryan Holland
Carleton Place

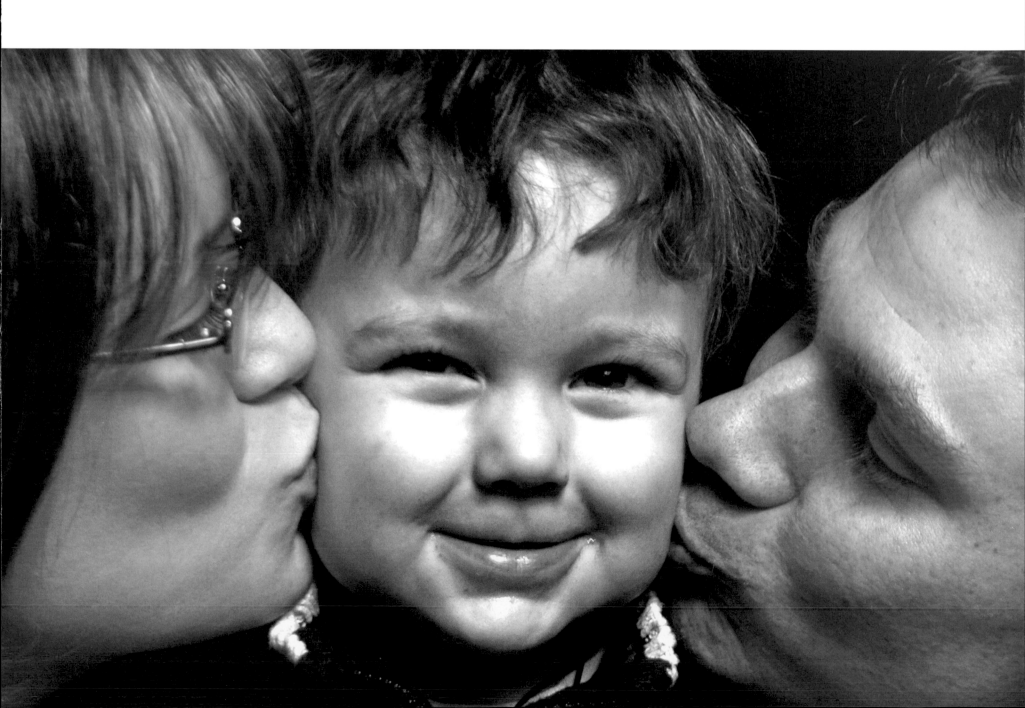

David

David Harris underwent four major surgeries for throat cancer. "I can't eat food, my speech is only partially intelligible, and three-quarters of my tongue has been replaced," he says. "I am a physical mess but lucky and appreciative to still be around. I figure, if there are women brave enough to expose their radical mastectomies, I can take my shirt off."

Photographer
David Harris
Utterson

Raymond

The photographer's father, Raymond Chen, was diagnosed with cancer of the nasopharynx at the age of 41. Six months of radiation destroyed the cancer as well as his salivary gland. Now 69, Raymond has lived to see the birth of his four grandchildren. His son says, "The cancer was life changing, yes; life ending, no. Go, Dad, go!"

Photographer
Roderick Chen
Markham

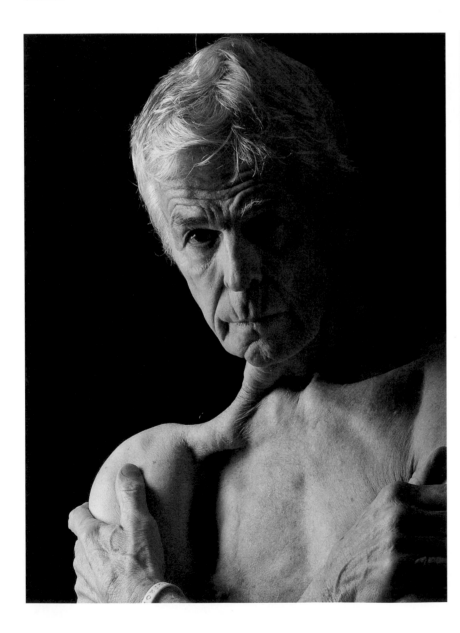

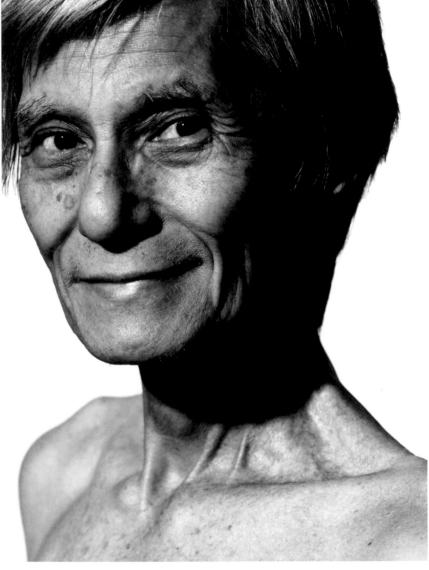

Kyle

Erika and Ryan of Rowell Photography are members of Smiling Eyes, a charity that offers free photo sessions to families living with cancer. At the beginning of the session, Kyle was very shy and hid behind a curtain until he felt ready to come out.

Photographers
Erika Hanchar and
Ryan Rowell
Sault Ste. Marie

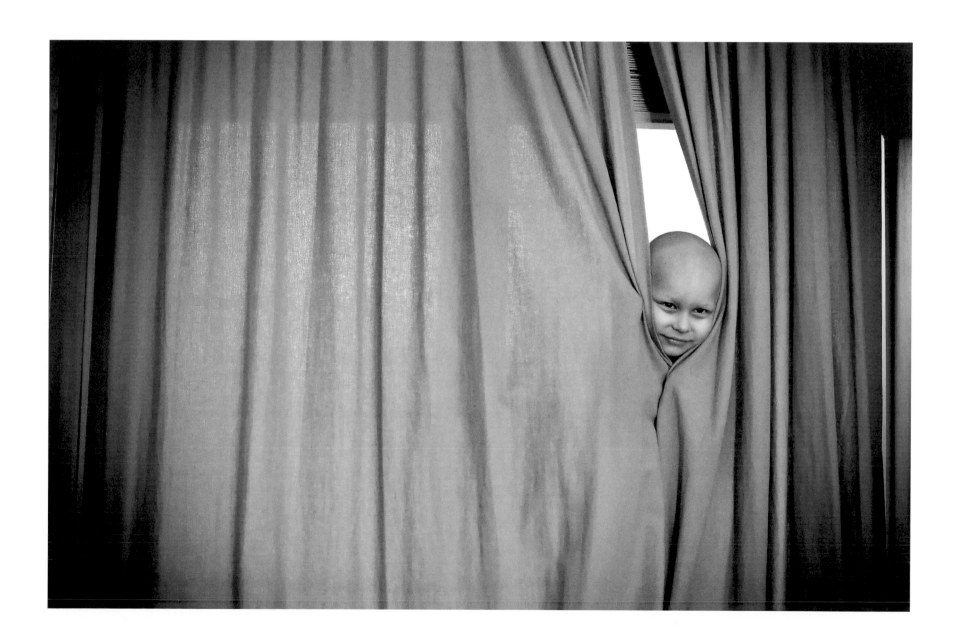

Earl

David Roth's father,
Earl, died of bone cancer
over 20 years ago. Each
time David knots his tie the
way his father showed
him, he is reminded of him.

Photographer
Vicky Roth
Cambridge

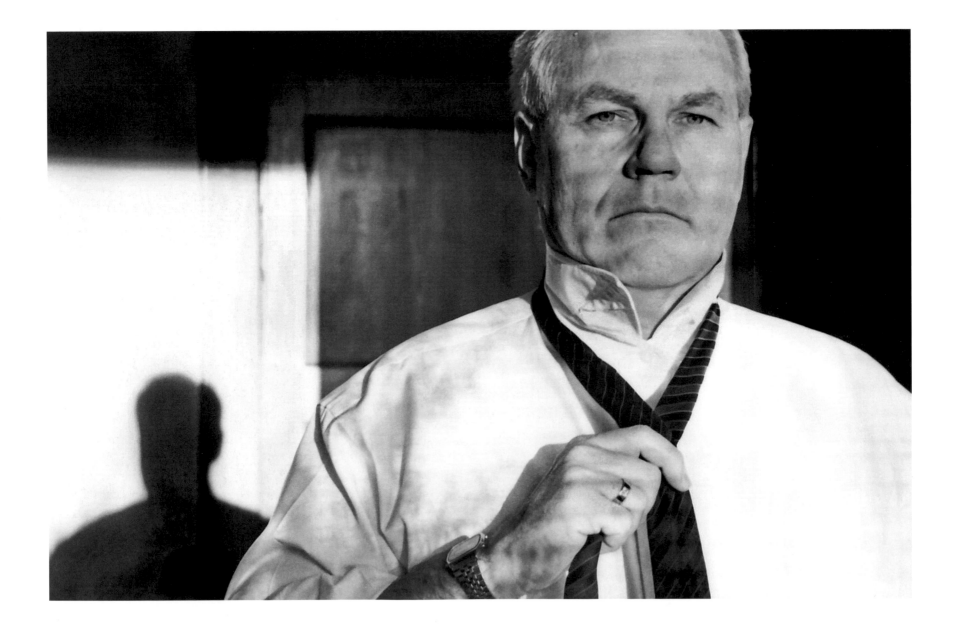

Shirley

Shirley Griffioen
was diagnosed with stage 1
breast cancer in 2003;
she had seven months of
treatment, which
included six rounds of
chemotherapy and 25 rounds
of radiation. She then joined
the "Busting Out" dragon
boat team.

Photographer
Judy Slack
Nepean

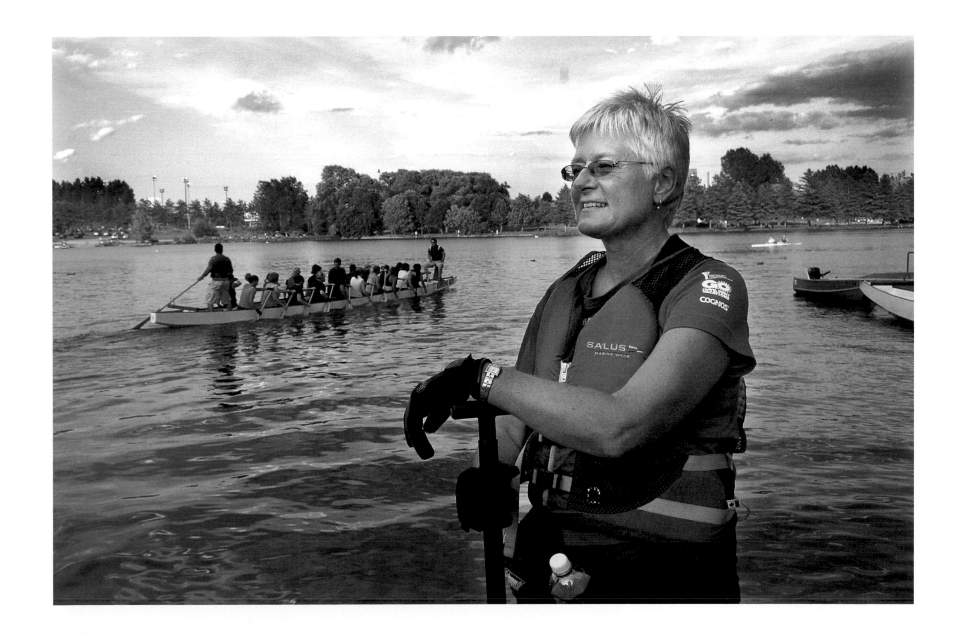

Dominique

Dominique Hebert on her horse Calypso. Dominique, a cancer survivor, says that Calypso has played a great part in her healing process, both before and after her cancer surgery.

Photographer
Fred Chartrand
Ottawa

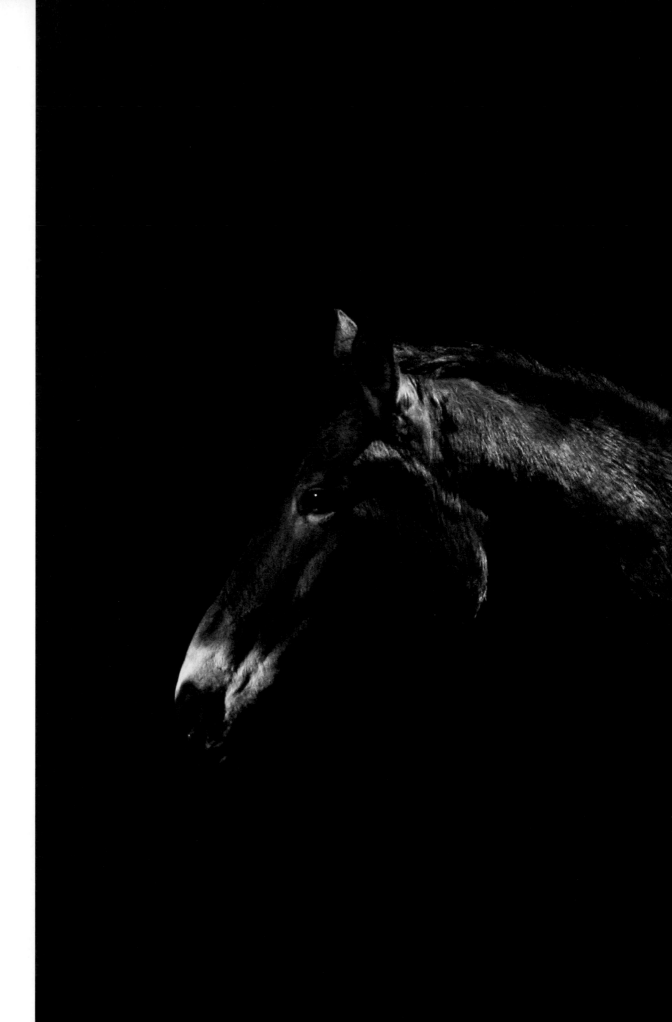

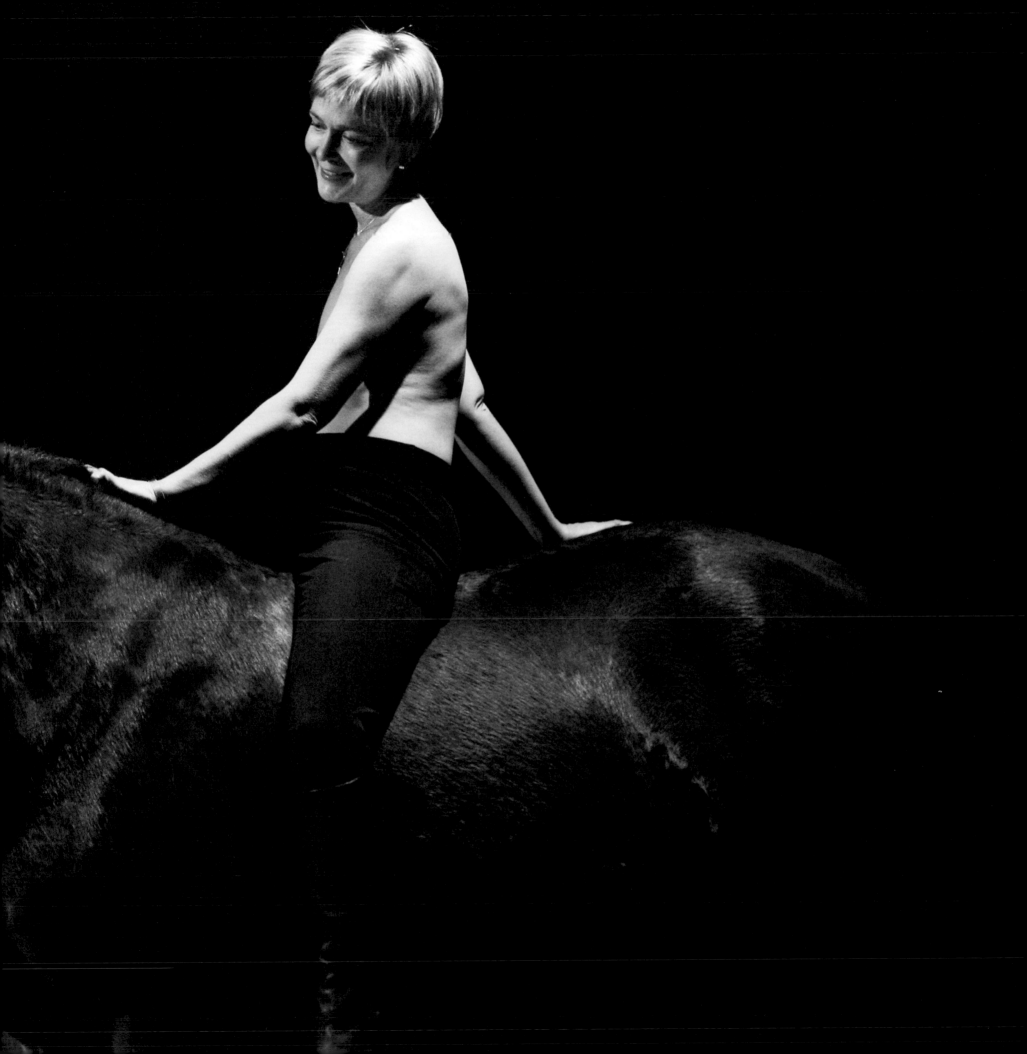

Yvonne

Yvonne McKenna, the photographer's mother, died at age 52 of breast cancer following four years of radical mastectomies and chemotherapy. Tim still remembers her smile and, though he can't recall the sound of her laugh, he says, "She laughed all the time." Her granddaughters Taryn (left), Katie (centre), and Lexi know her only through stories and photos.

Photographer
Tim McKenna
Oakville

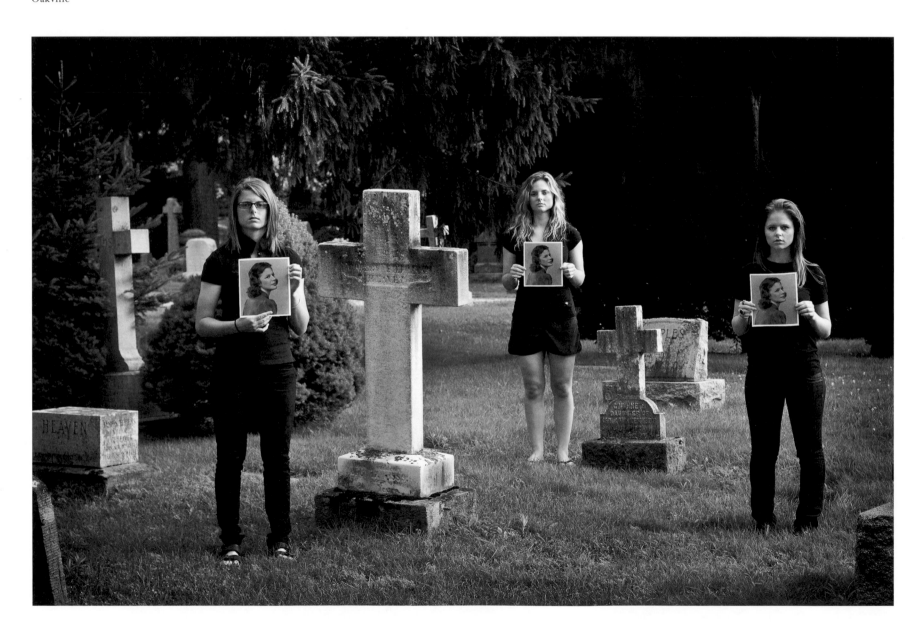

"What I love about my mother

are her smile and laugh. Her laugh lifts

my spirit, her smile radiates love."

Alan Joson

Tammy

Tammy Cote (far right) with her family while on a vacation in PEI. A year earlier, Tammy had undergone chemotherapy for leukemia, and by the time of the vacation, she was in remission. Tammy says "It symbolizes our great joy at being cancer-free and back to normal, everyday life."

Photographer
Danielle Perry Curran

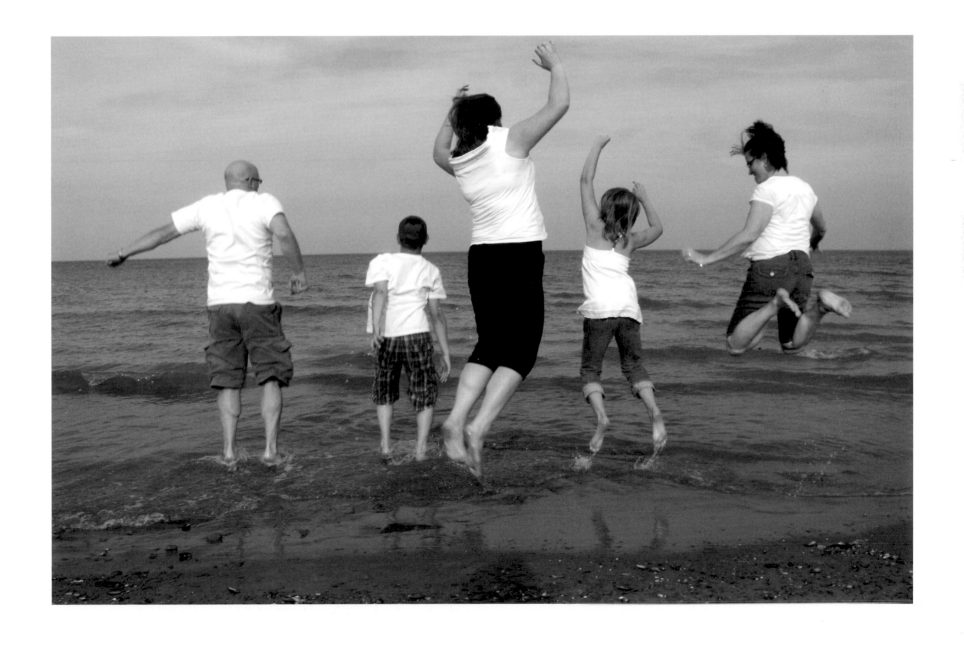

Carmel

Carmel Darmanin with
Mary, his wife. Carmel is
a two-time cancer survivor;
he fought colon cancer
and is now recovering from
lung cancer.

Photographer
Jessica Darmanin
Woodbridge

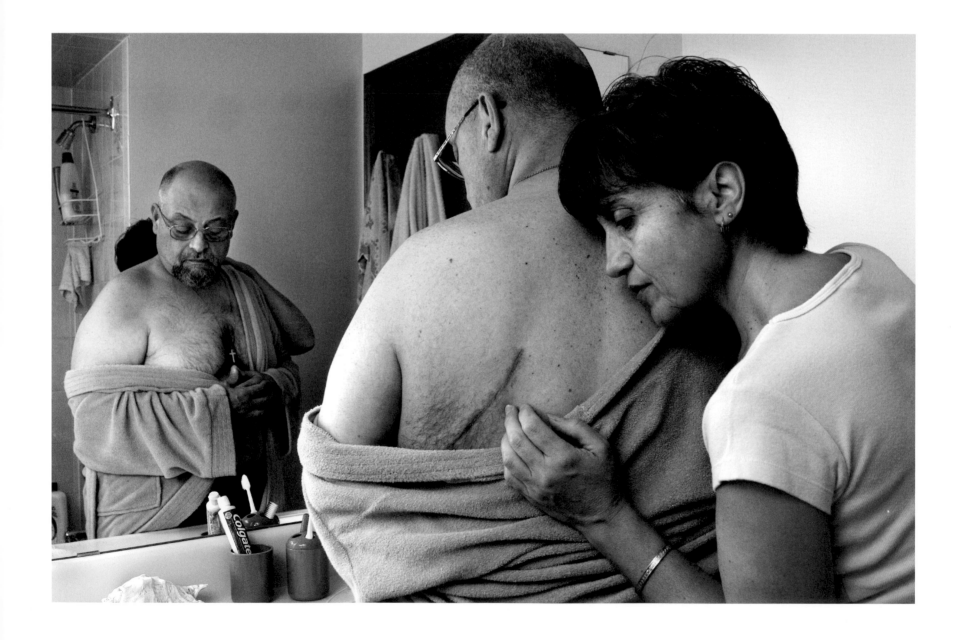

Yael

The photographer's wife, Yael Boening, was first diagnosed with breast cancer in 1998. In 2001, cancer was found in her other breast and Yael decided on a double mastectomy. In 2008, the cancer spread to her bones, skull, and liver. Yael and her team of doctors are still fighting the disease.

Photographer
Patrick Boening
Richmond Hill

Peggy

Peggy Tripp is remarkable in having survived four different types of cancer; breast, bone, and Hodgkin's and non-Hodgkin's lymphoma. During each chemotherapy treatment, her husband Wayne shaves his head to show his love and support. She has been diagnosed with a fifth cancer and plans to fight it, too.

Photographer
Lori Fox-Rossi
Thunder Bay

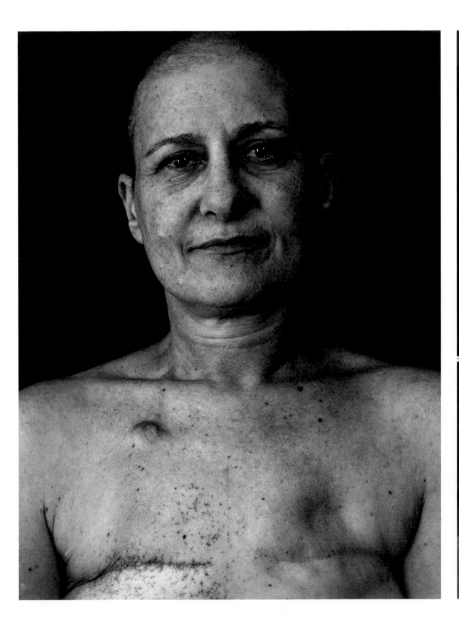

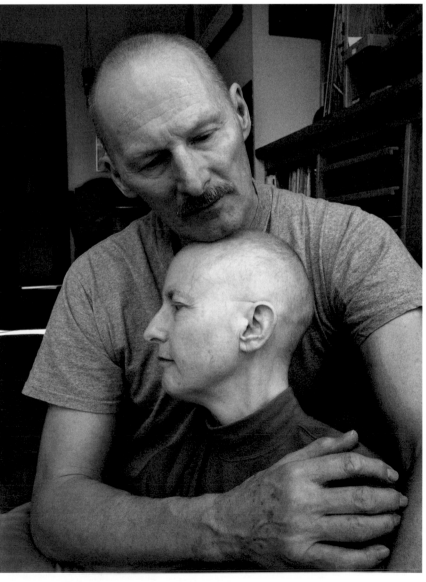

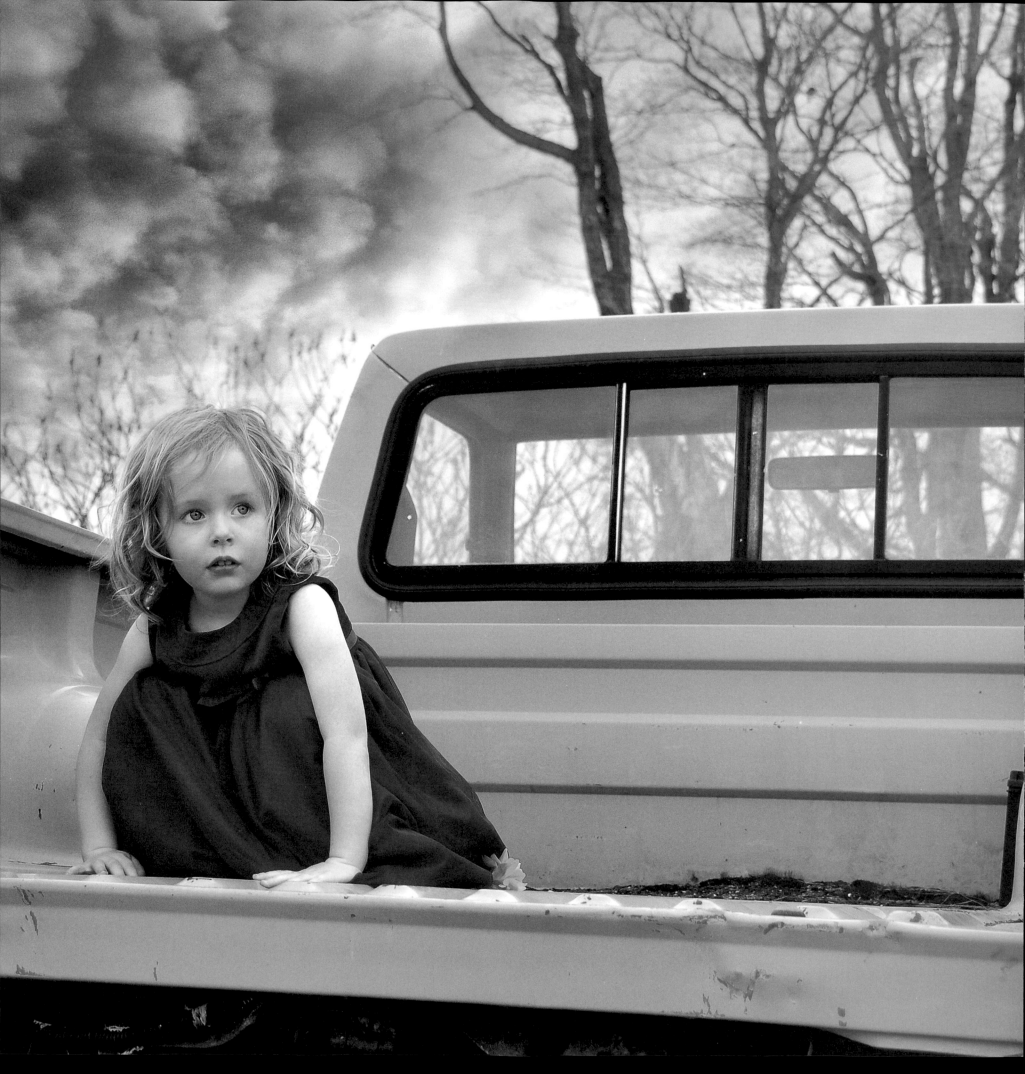

Photographer
Jennifer Gillespie
Waterloo

Breanna

Breanna Gillespie-Bumstead was only 17 months old when she suddenly developed a high fever, started vomiting and coughing, and became very lethargic. Her mother, photographer Jennifer Gillespie, knew that something was seriously wrong with her.

"I thought she had pneumonia," says Jennifer. "When the doctor told me to just give her Tylenol, I knew in my heart that it was something worse than a cold."

Ignoring the doctor's advice, and with her 10-week-old son Trevor in tow, Jennifer took Breanna to the emergency unit of her local hospital. Doctors checked Breanna's vital signs and discovered that she had restricted breathing. They took an X-ray, which revealed a large tumour in her chest.

"It was neuroblastoma," says Jennifer, "one of the most aggressive cancers. I was still thinking it was pneumonia. I usually think that everything in life happens for a reason, but this was the only time when I thought, 'What can be the reason for this? What child deserves to have cancer?'"

Breanna was immediately transferred to the Hospital for Sick Children in Toronto, where surgeons opened up her back to take the tumour out. "We were very lucky," Jennifer says. "Neuroblastoma can spread to other parts of the body and be deadly. Surgery was enough for Breanna. She didn't even need to have chemotherapy or radiation."

Nevertheless, the three weeks that the family spent at the hospital were nightmarish. "At one point my mother-in-law told me to get some sleep," Jennifer remembers. "But I didn't want to fall asleep, because then I would wake up and realize it wasn't all just a bad dream."

Although Breanna was given a very good prognosis after the surgery, it took a long time for Jennifer to believe it and feel that her daughter was going to be OK. "I can really relate to people with post-traumatic stress. The whole experience really hit me hard."

Breanna is now four and a healthy, happy little girl. "I now look at it as a blessing in disguise," says Jennifer. "There are so many positives. After Breanna got sick, I wanted to capture every moment I could with her. I got a good camera, it became a passion, and now I am a professional photographer."

Jennifer and her husband Chris have also spent a lot of time over the last few years raising thousands of dollars for the Hospital for Sick Children, participating in marathons and in the Iron Man. "Breanna has been healthy for three years so that is all in the past for us. Now it's all about helping the other kids who aren't so fortunate."

Evelyn

Evelyn Joson was diagnosed with uterine cancer in 1994. She had a hysterectomy on her son Alan's birthday and has been cancer-free since. Alan says, "What I love about my mother are her smile and laugh. Her laugh lifts my spirit, her smile radiates love."

Photographer
Alan Joson
Scarborough

Jack

Jack Woolley, touring around the hospital, with his favourite iced coffee, escorted by his grand-daughter, Lindsay Worboys. Jack enjoyed life to the fullest, golfing and dancing into his last year. Metastatic cancer was diagnosed in his spine days after his 91st Christmas in 2009. One possible primary source was lymphoma, but that was never confirmed before he passed away a month later.

Photographer
Nikki Wesley
Mississauga

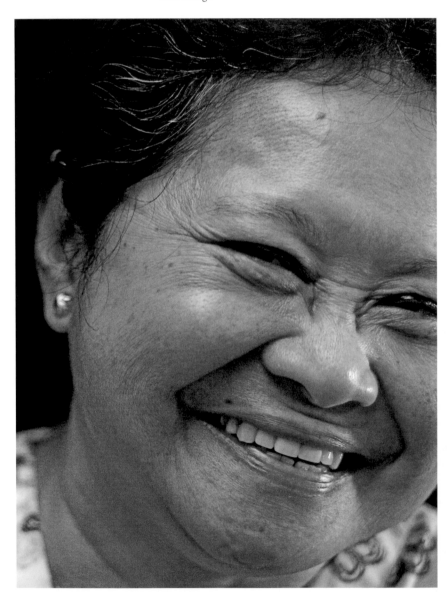

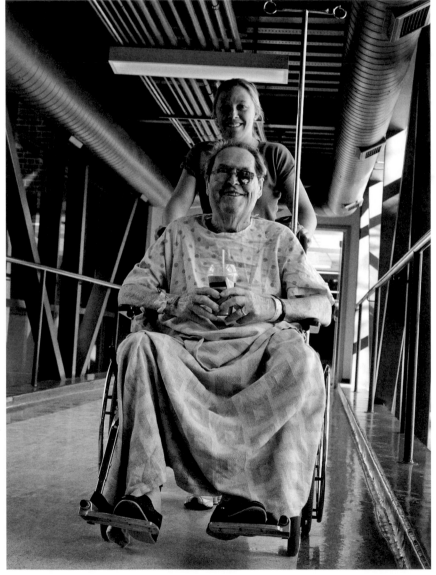

Cheryl

A breast cancer survivor, Cheryl Jackson found the location for the photo shoot to be very appropriate. "It incorporates the beauty of the lake and the serenity it gives us cancer survivors as we progress through the healing process," she says.

Photographer
Tom Thomson
Kenora

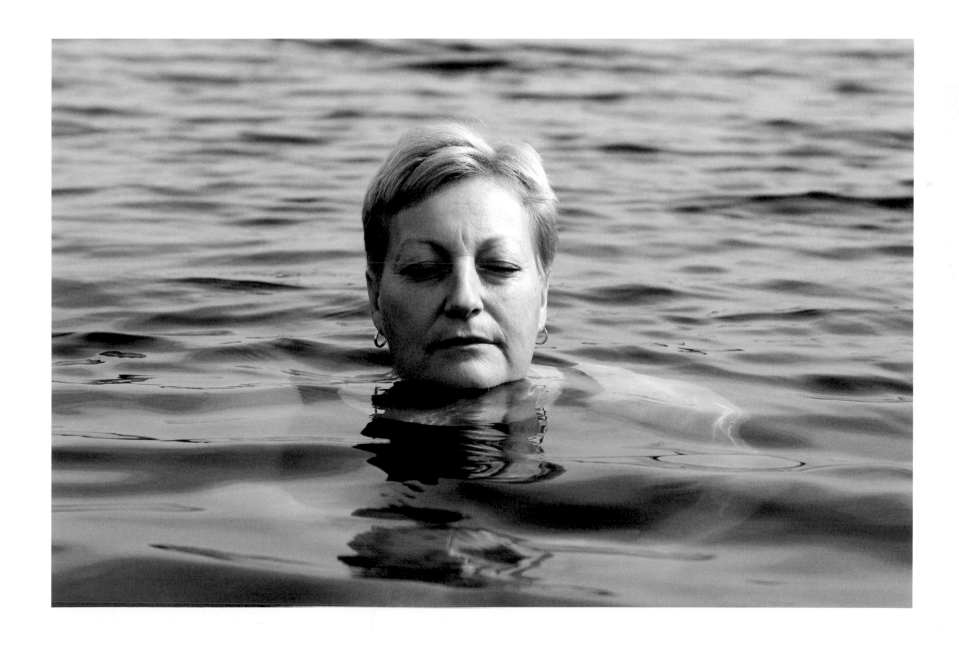

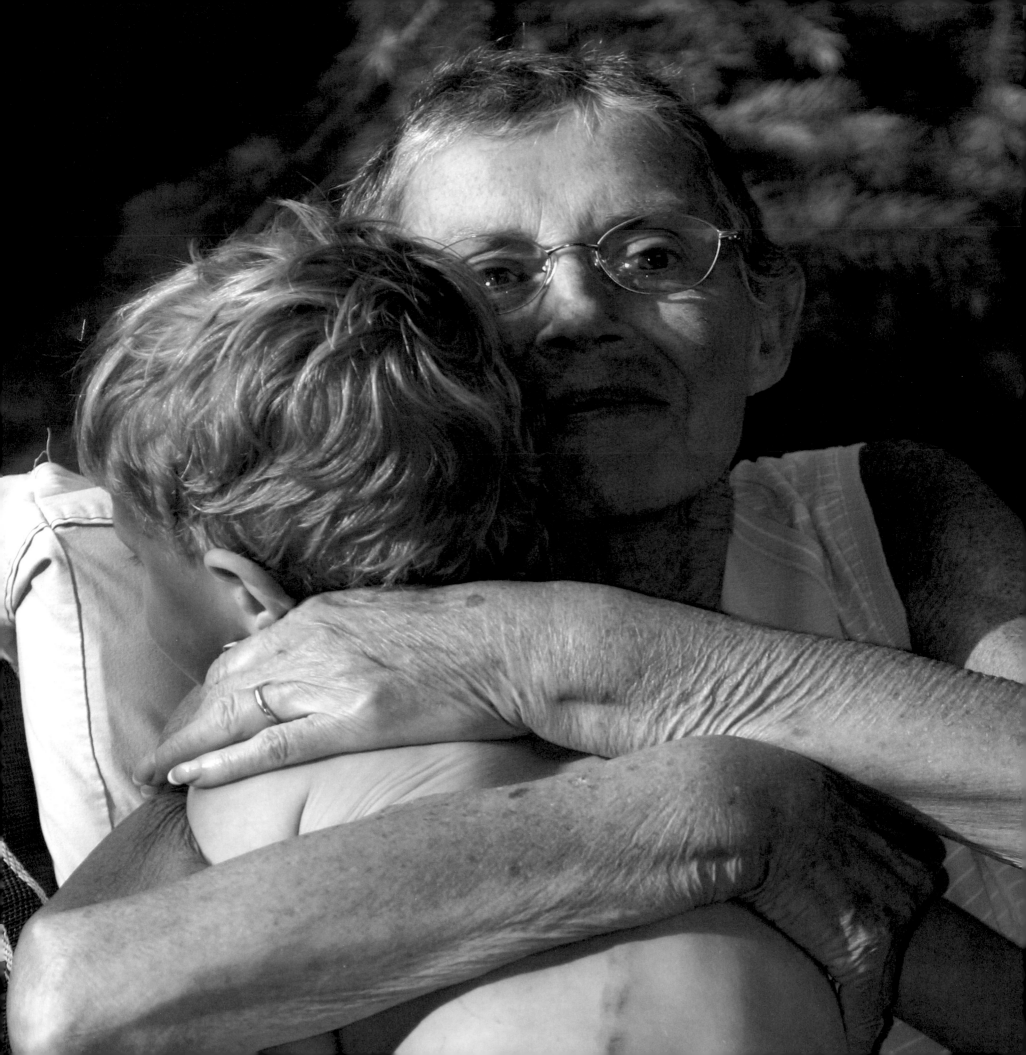

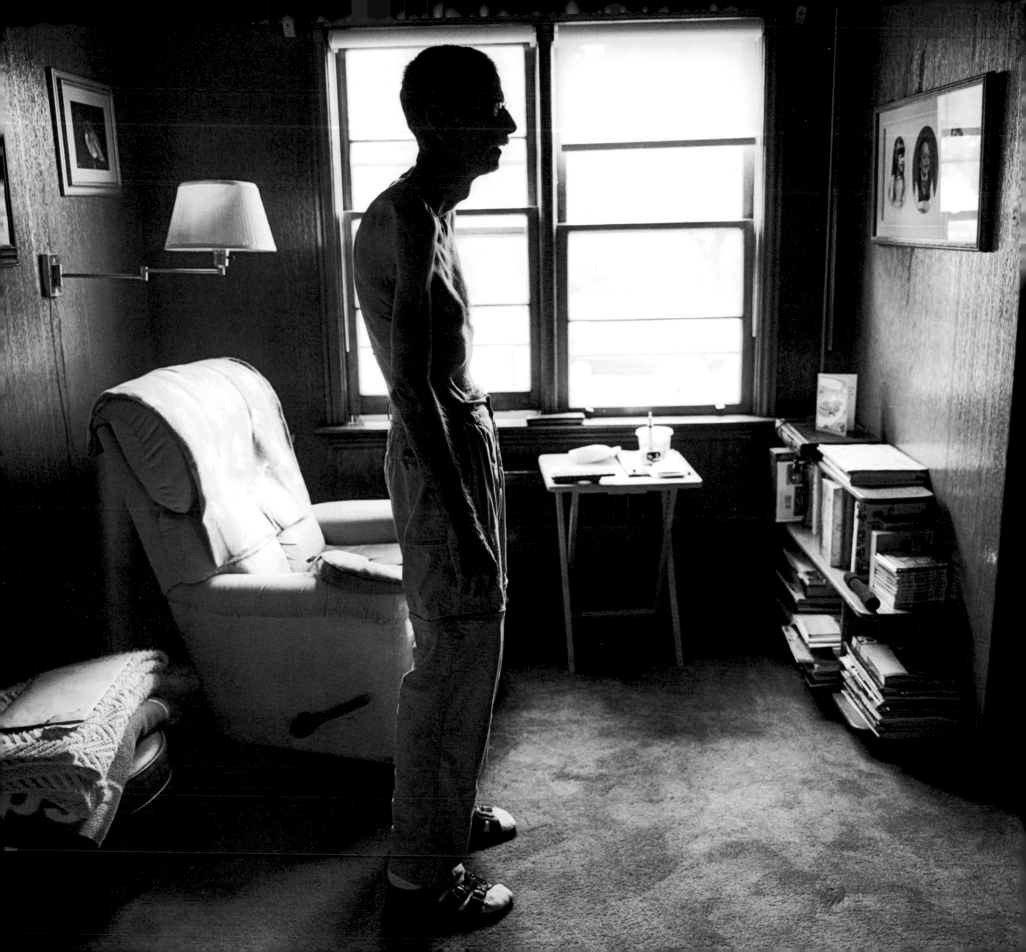

Previous left

Cynthia

Cynthia Wittick, suffering from esophageal cancer, embraces her grandson Carter. Despite undergoing chemotherapy and radiation, the cancer spread to Cynthia's liver and brain, and she died seven weeks after this image was captured.

Photographer
Cameron Wittick
Willowdale

Previous right

Blayne

The late Blayne Kinart, a former chemical worker who suffered from mesothelioma, a form of cancer associated with exposure to asbestos. Blayne worked at a chemical plant in Sarnia, Ontario, where he was frequently exposed to asbestos for most of his working career.

Photographer
Louie Palu
Sarnia

Kaye

Kaye Brown and her son Richard share a moment with a portrait of her husband, whom they lost to pancreatic cancer. He was diagnosed only five days before he died.

Photographer
Farzana Wahidy
Belleville

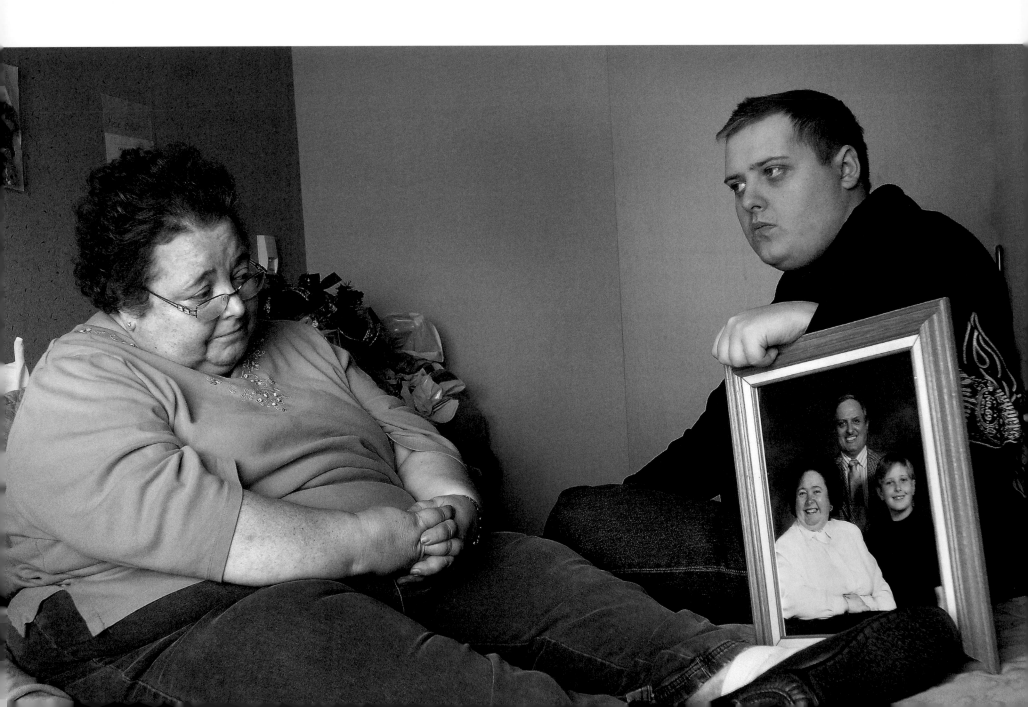

Doug

Photographer Valerie Rempel had had a difficult relationship with her stepfather Doug Chambers. However, when both of Valerie's sons were born with serious illnesses, Doug begged God to take him instead of them. Doug died of lung cancer and both boys made full recoveries. Valerie says, "Illness can tear a family apart, but in my case it brought us together."

Photographer
Valerie Rempel
Brights Grove

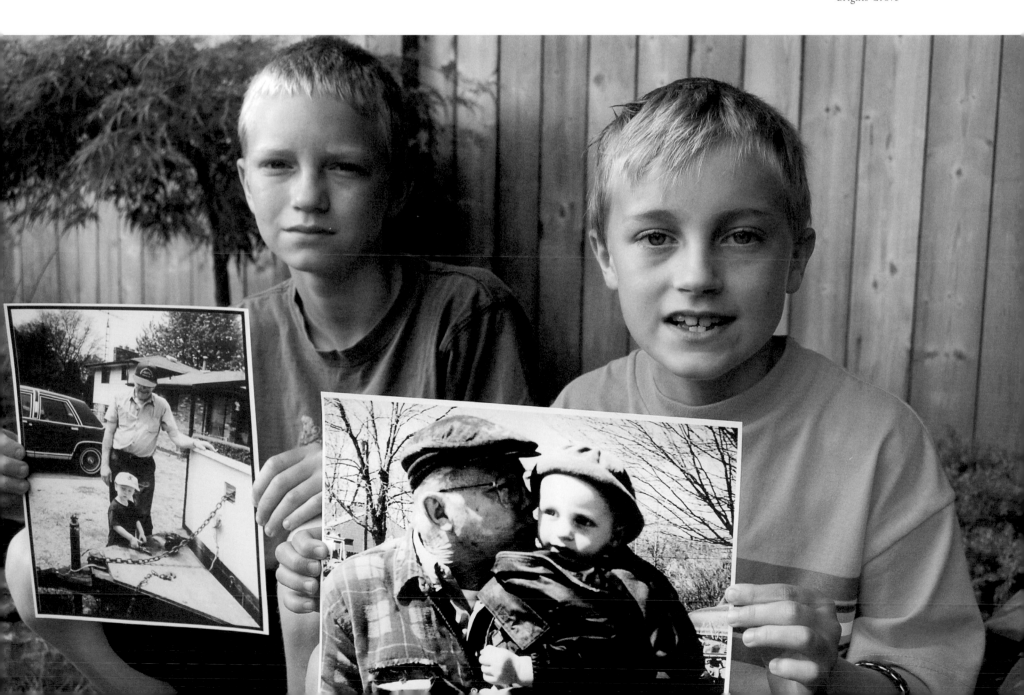

Ryan

Ryan Allan, 24, says there isn't a day that passes without him thinking about his mother, who passed away in 2004 from leukemia and lymphoma.

Photographer
Karen Neff
Kingston

Nathan

Nathan's father, Captain Bob Shaw, a firefighter in Hamilton, Ontario, gave his life so others could have theirs. He made the ultimate sacrifice, dying as the result of a toxic fire, which caused the cancer that took his life. "I witnessed his strength, courage, and determination in the face of unimaginable adversity," says Nathan. "I lost my dad, my best friend, my hero."

Photographer
Simon Wilson
Hamilton

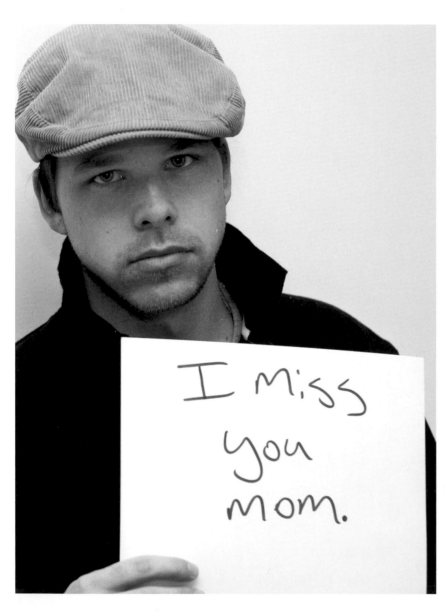

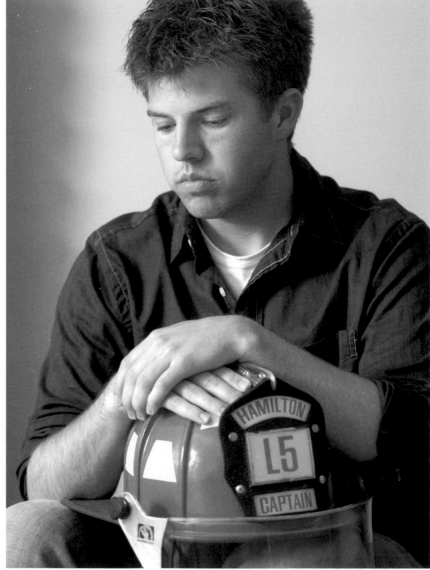

Over

Dan

The photographer took this image of her Uncle Dan, who had a passion for cooking, sitting peacefully in his kitchen in December 2007. He was receiving chemotherapy, having been diagnosed with colon cancer four months earlier. Sadly, he passed away in March 2008.

Photographer
Kendra Vamplew
Oakville

John

John "Jet" Leslie of Arnprior, Ontario, lost his leg to osteosarcoma. Today, at 16, John plays for the Canadian U18 Amputee Hockey Team.

Photographer
Mike Pochwat
Arnprior

Angela

"Inner Solace: self-portrait of a chemo patient." The photographer is a breast cancer survivor.

Photographers
Angela Merrett
Woodbridge

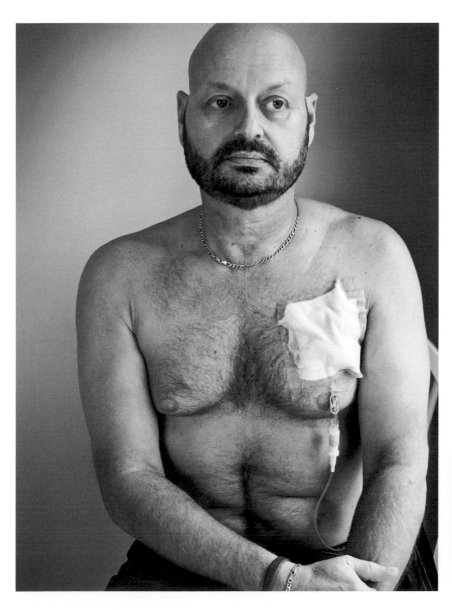

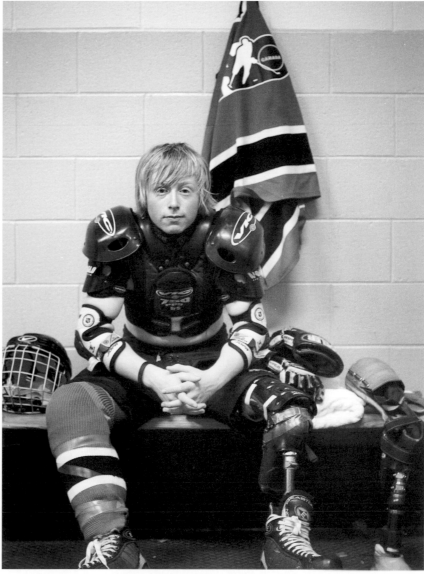

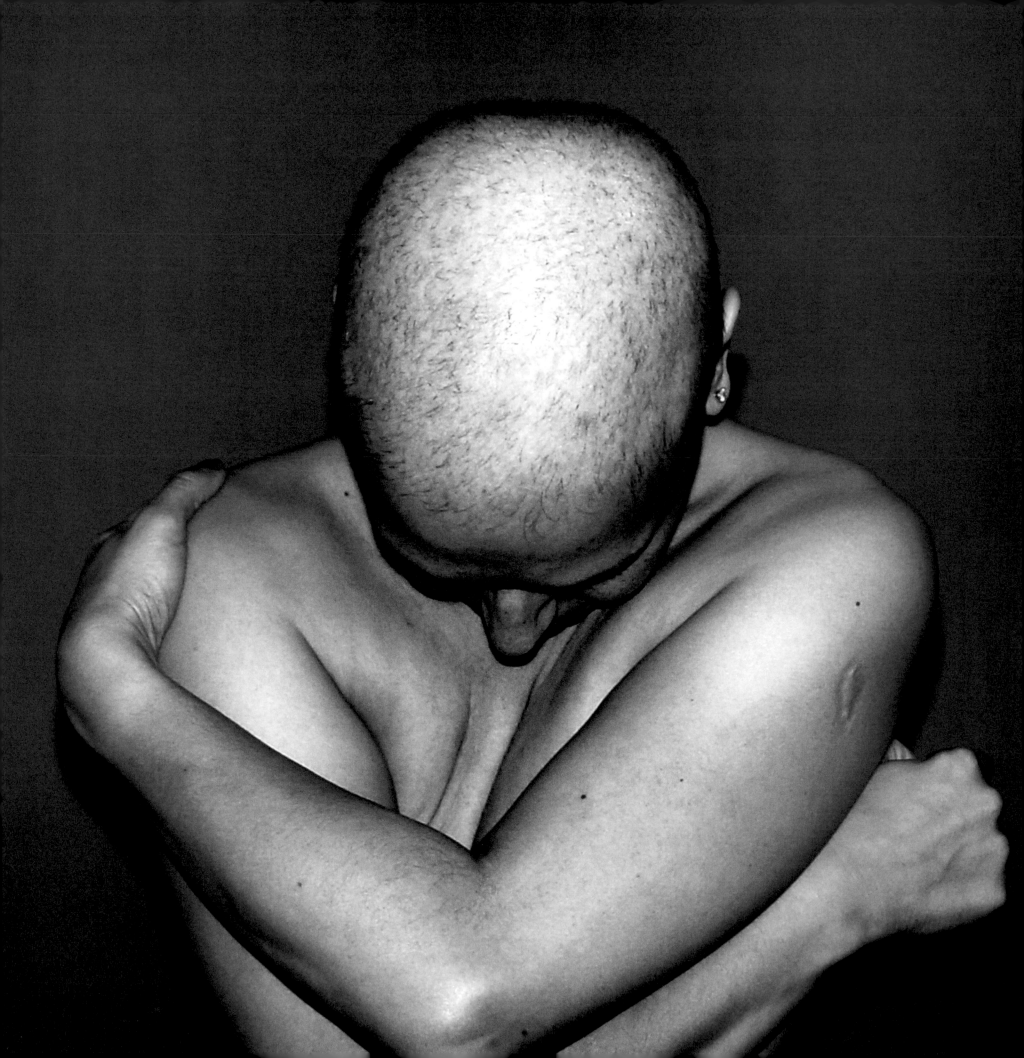

Row 1: Aaron Whitfield, Pickering; Alex Lainson, Cambridge; Alex Mackie (3–4), Stittsville; Alexandra Stephanson, Picton; Ali Thompson, Oakville; Allan Rock, Ottawa; Amber Wilson, Peterborough

Row 2: Amber Soroka, Roseville; Andrea Raymond, Brampton; Andrew Stawicki, Mississauga; Angele Cote (4–5), Curran; Anne Moser, Mississauga; Arthur Uyeyama, Mississauga; Bethany Sanders, Cambridge

Row 3: Bethany Sanders, Cambridge; Bill Grimshaw (2–3), Port Carling; Brian Summers, Port Perry; Brian Summers, Little Britain; Brian Barrer, Barrie; Brianne Bassett, Stittsville; Bryan Davies, Creemore

Row 4: Bryan Davies, Corbetton; Cece Scott, Mississauga; Caitlin den Boer, Burlington; Camille Talag, Whitby; Carol Cooper, Thunder Bay; Casey Lessard, Grand Bend; Cathy Chatterton, Douro; Chris Mikula, Ottawa

Row 5: Chris Bumstead, Waterloo; Christine Bracewell, Essex; Christine Kufske (3–4), Waterloo; Clare Geddes, Cambridge; Constance Legg, London; Courtney Payne, Mississauga; Courtney Butler, Cambridge

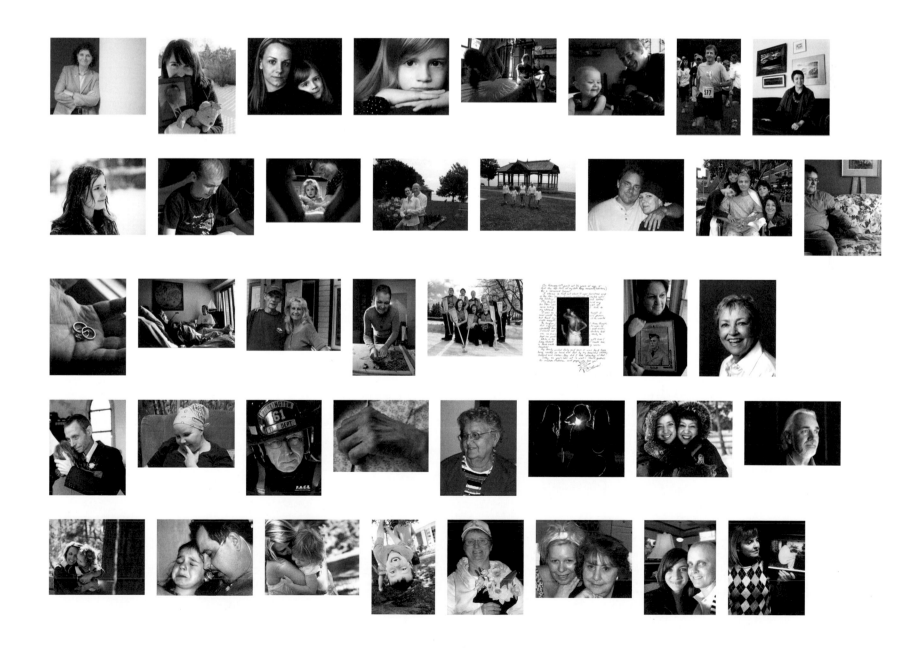

Row 1: Dimitri Stippelmans, Cayuga; Daniel Vendramin, Scarborough; Dave Chidley (3–8), London

Row 2: David Hou, Conn; David Porter, Richmond Hill; David Richer-Brulé (3–5), Ottawa; Deb Ransom, Ottawa; Derek Cassidy, Belleville; Dimitra Perentesis, London

Row 3: Dinah Ener, Cornwall; Don Mallory, Hamilton; Donna Santos (3–5), Brampton; Elise von Kulmiz, Scarborough; Elizabeth Siegfried, Dwight; Elisha Souto, Cambridge

Row 4: Elliot Ferguson, Woodstock; Eric St-Amant, Ottawa; Erica Barton, Kingston; Erika Hanchar and Ryan Rowell (4–6), Sault Ste. Marie; Erin Keller (7–8), Richmond Hill

Row 5: Erin Samuel, Baden; Fern Blais (2–3), Pembroke; Frank Mazzuca, Kleinburg; Frank Mazzuca, North York; Frank O'Connor, Belleville; G. Szeto, Richmond Hill; Gary Bate, Garson

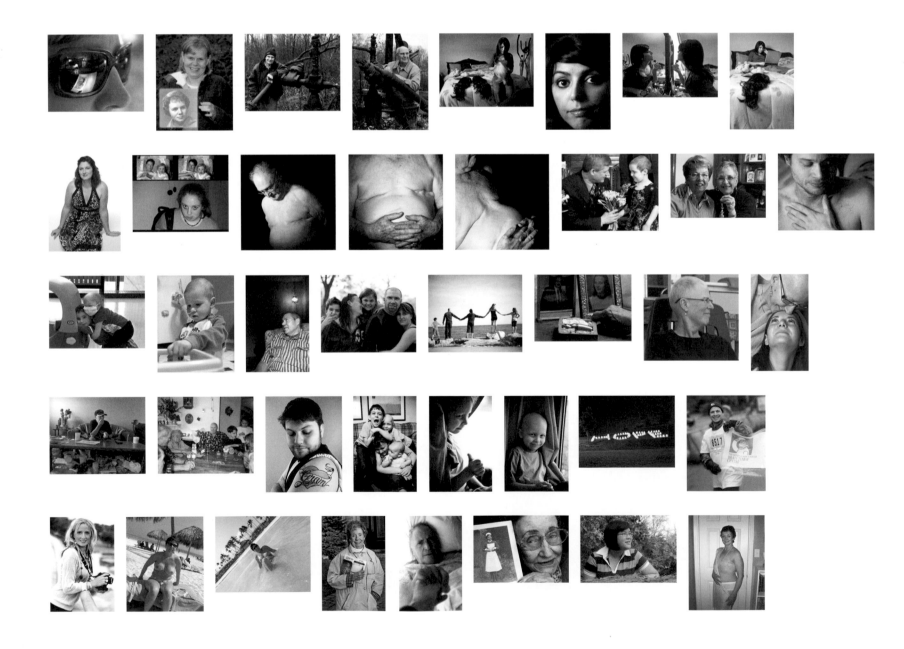

Row 1: Graham Eby, Cambridge; Grant Kennedy, Ottawa; Gregory Yapp (3–4), Thornhill; Hannah Desmarais, Cambridge; Heather Wiebe, Belleville; Heather Rivet (7–8), Orillia

Row 2: Heather Rivet (1–2), Orillia; Hugh Wesley (3–4), Burlington; Ian Wilson, Amherstview; Ian James Hopkins, Ottawa; Irina Souiki (7–8), Newmarket

Row 3: Irina Souiki, Newmarket; Jamie Diamond, (2–4), Richmond Hill; Janie Laird, Ajax; Jean Boulay (6–7), Ottawa; Jeff Boyce, Belleville

Row 4: Jennifer Globush, Balmertown; Jennifer Gillespie (2–5), Waterloo; Jesse Foster, London; Jessica Montroy, Cornwall; Jessica Mulholland, Belleville

Row 5: Jo-Ann McArthur (1–4), Perth; Jodi Pembleton, Mississauga; Joe Pace, Oshawa; John Fearnall, Owen Sound; John Gaudi, Wiarton

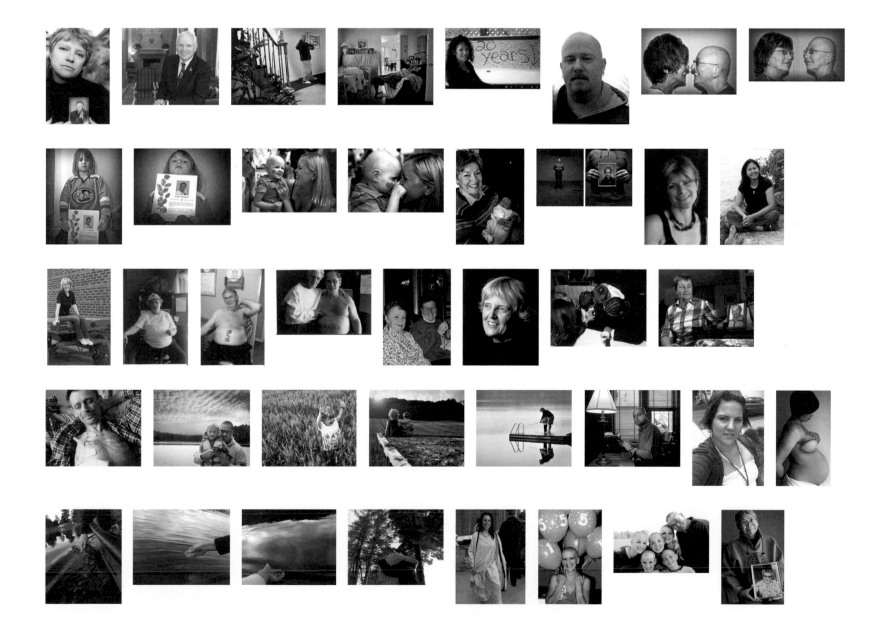

Row 1: John McNally, Belle River; Joy Timleck, Brampton; Julie Nyree, Mississauga; Kali Rees, Cambridge; Karen Perlmutter, Thornhill; Karen Wray, London; Katie Wiesel, Cambridge; Katy McDonald, Oakville

Row 2: Kelly Davidson, Ottawa; Kelly Wilk, Newmarket; Kelly Williams, Burlington; Kevin Spreekmeester, Mississauga; Krista Messier, Cambridge; Kristi Rajala, Mississauga; Kristina Laukkanen, Scarborough; Larry Frank, Brantford

Row 3: Larry Frank, Brantford; Lars Hagberg (2–4), Inverary; Laura Bombier (5–7), Huntsville; Leah Durrer, Cambridge

Row 4: Lisa Graves, L'Orignal; Liz Roberts, Picton; Lori Eagleson, Ottawa; Luciana Nechita, Windsor; Marilyn Walsh, Palmerston; Mark Spowart, London; Martin Ranger, Burlington; Mary Jane MacVicar, Leamington

Row 5: Mary Jane MacVicar, Leamington; Megan Peterson, Waterloo; Meghan Niittynen, Thunder Bay; Melanie Green, Mississauga; Melissa Munroe, Barrie; Menno Meijer, London; Michele Taras (7–8), Brampton

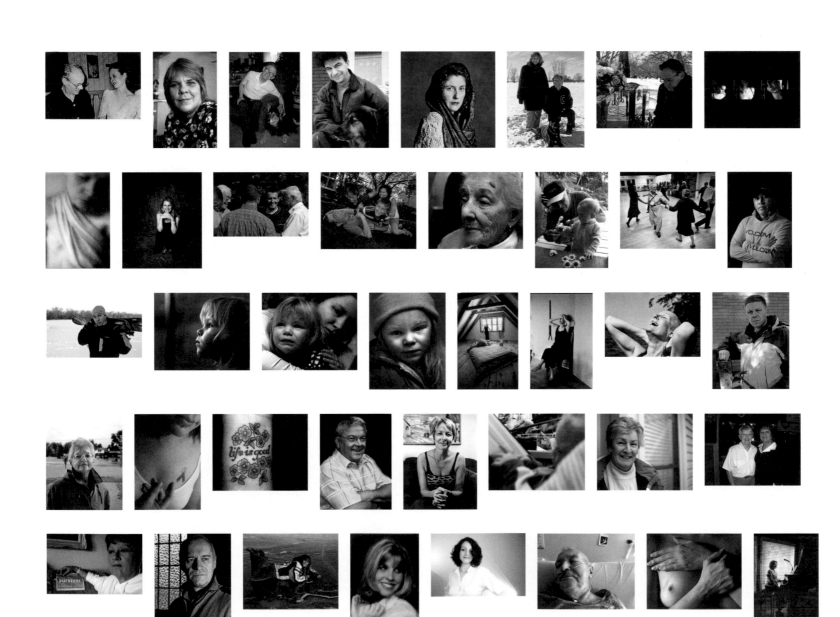

Row 1: Michele Taras (1–8), Brampton

Row 2: Michele Taras (1–8), Brampton

Row 3: Michele Taras (1–3), Brampton; Michelle Blais, Pembroke; Mirko Petricevic (5–6), Kitchener; Molly McNulty, Belleville; Monica McKenna, Sunderland

Row 4: Nancy Coull, Scarborough; Natalie Volpe, Cambridge; Natasha Fillion, Ottawa; Nikki Wesley, Mississauga; Nina Vogel, Cambridge; Owen Wong, Scarborough; Patrick Byers, Oshawa; Patrick J. Boehing, Richmond Hill

Row 5: Patte Foreman (1–2), Thunder Bay; Paul Walker, Oakville; Paul Walker, Mississauga; Paul Walker, Melbourne; Paul Yelle, Mississauga; Pauline Szczesniak, Kitchener; Peter Bregg, Ottawa

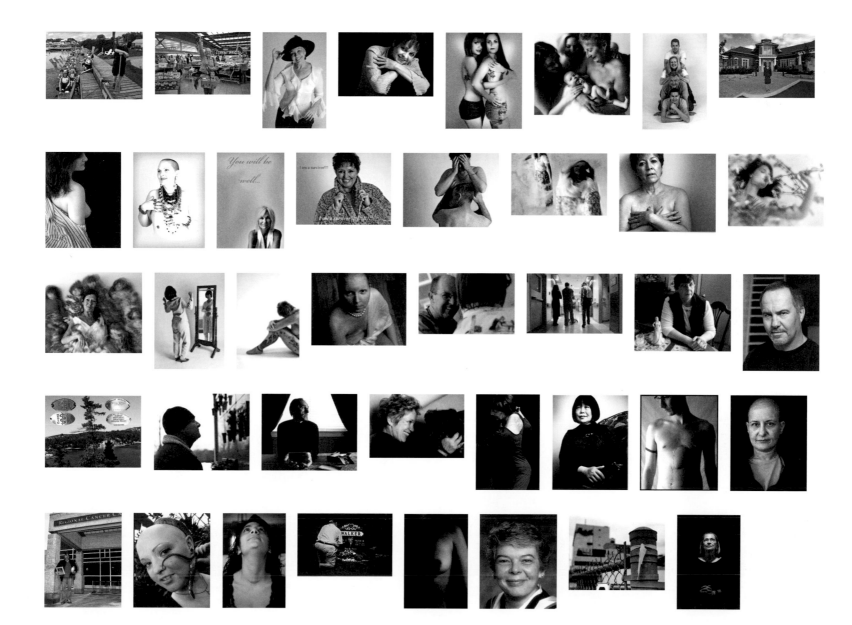

Row 1: Peter Bregg, Ottawa; Peter Mason, Renfrew; R. Dale Copeland, Colborne; Ray Pilon, Ottawa; Renato Rossi, Mississauga; René Calderón, Kingston; Richard Brown, North York; Richard Kropman, Thornhill

Row 2: Robert Shannon, Aurora; Roberto Varela, Brampton; Ron Bernardo, Hamilton; Rozemarijn Oudejans, Ottawa; Salina Kassam, Mississauga; Sandra Regier, Exeter; Sandy Ziegler, Ottawa; Sarah Corbett, Orangeville

Row 3: Shanna Larsen, Woodstock; Shannon Maguire, Orono; Sharon Erlichman, Thornhill; Sharon M. Ross, London; Shayla Snobelen, Cambridge; Simon Bell (6–7), Guelph; Spencer Adams, Kitchener

Row 4: Susan Ashukian, St. Catharines; Susan Bate, Garson; Suzanne Williams (3–4), Mississauga; Suzanne Robertson, Perth; Suzy Lamont, Kingston; Tarin Mead, Red Lake; Teresa Olson, Richmond Hill

Row 5: Teresa Olson (1–2), Richmond Hill; Tina Martins, Whitby; Tom Dykstra, Ottawa; Tom Thomson (5–8), Kenora

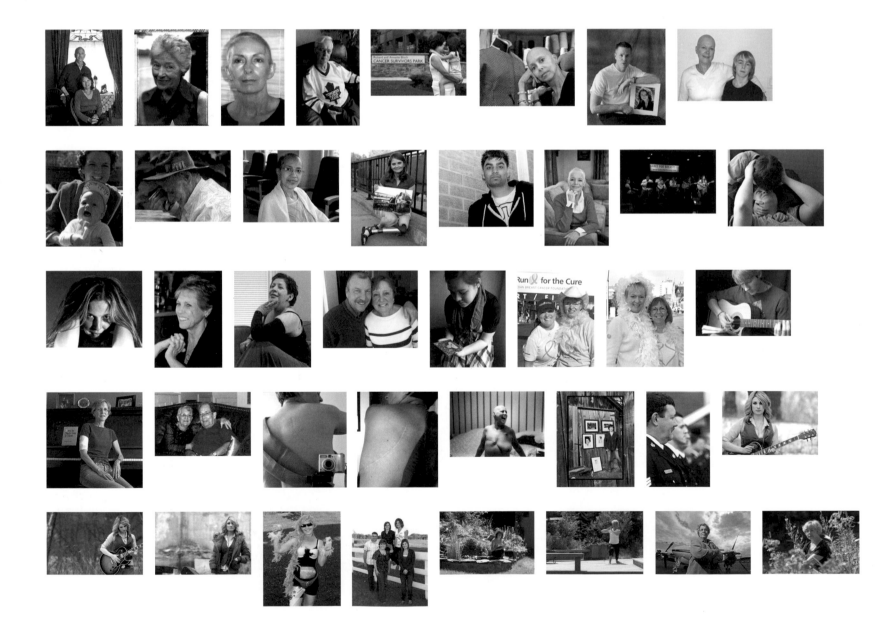

Row 1: Tom Thomson (1–8), Kenora

Row 2: Tom Thomson (1–4), Kenora; V. Tony Hauser (5–6), Ottawa, Ajax; Tory Zimmerman, Caledon; Travis Allison, Woodstock

Row 3: Travis Allison (1–4), Woodstock; Ute Bruno, Brantford; Valerie Rempel (6–8), Brights Grove, Sarnia

Row 4: Valerie Rempel (1–8), Brights Grove, Sarnia

Row 5: Valerie Rempel (1–2), Brights Grove, Sarnia; Vicky Roth, Cambridge; Victoria Harris, Cambridge; Virginia Macdonald, Mississauga; Wayne Cuddington, Ottawa

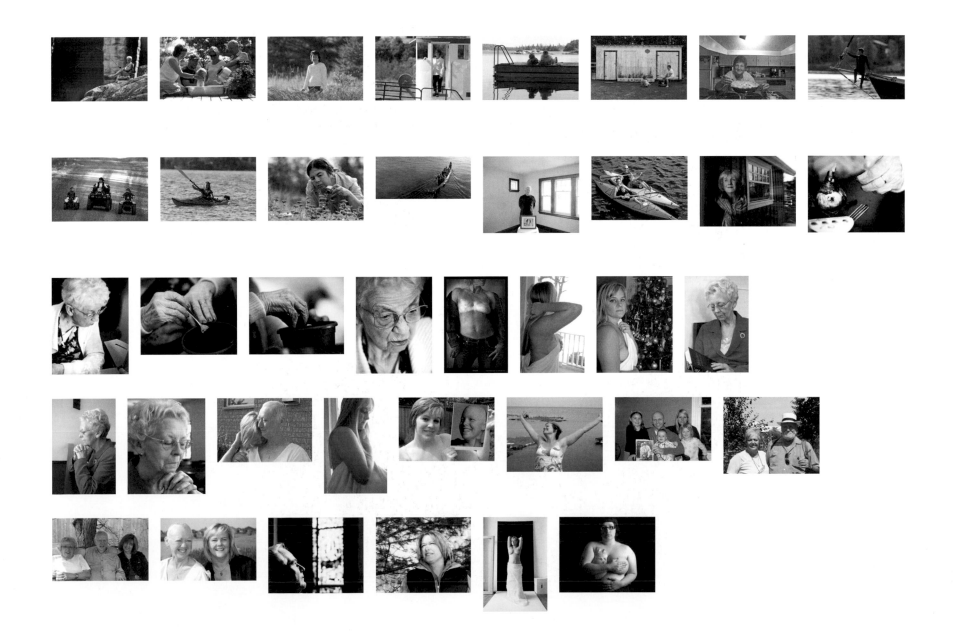

Toronto

"Live life to the fullest. The race is long and in the end it is only with yourself."

Margarida

Photographer
Sandra Smith
Toronto

Barbara

In 2006, Barbara Gadacz discovered that she had glycogen rich clear cell carcinoma, an extremely rare form of breast cancer. She also discovered that she was at stage 4 and that her prognosis was decidedly poor.

In 2008, Barbara submitted this photo to *Cancer Connections*. By this point, she had undergone a double mastectomy and intense chemotherapy and radiation. The marks that are visible on her chest are where the radiation had charred her skin.

"One in eight women will get breast cancer, but only 1 per cent of them will get my diagnosis," Barbara said. "It's that rare. So there's no research. No drug trials. Nothing. The doctors just had to blast me with everything in their arsenal to try to slow down my death. That's unconscionable. Every person and every cancer counts."

In spite of this grim reality, Barbara refused to give up the fight. She was also determined to help others in the same situation. When the Canadian Cancer Society asked to interview her on camera as part of their Fight Back campaign, she leapt at the chance. In the video, she was realistic but incredibly defiant.

Addressing her cancer, she said, "You keep coming after me, in my dreams. Over and over. But I get up every morning and I appreciate every single day. I will be the winner in this fight. Just like the way water takes down a mountain, I am going to take you down."

Unfortunately, Barbara's strength and immense courage couldn't prevent the cancer from spreading to her lungs, vertebrae, and rib cage. She still refused to give in: "I told the doctors, do whatever you have to do. Take me to the very edge of death and then pull me back."

In early 2010, the disease had taken such a strong hold that Barbara was admitted to palliative care at the Princess Margaret Hospital in Toronto. At that time, and in her typically selfless fashion, Barbara chose not to speak about herself, but rather the wonderful treatment she was receiving.

"While cancer is slowly robbing me of my health and my life, palliative care is where I am glad to be. It's all about making you feel comfortable. It's not a death-sentence place, it's about the living. And I am going to continue fighting with the last breath I have."

Barbara gave her last breath on May 21, 2010.

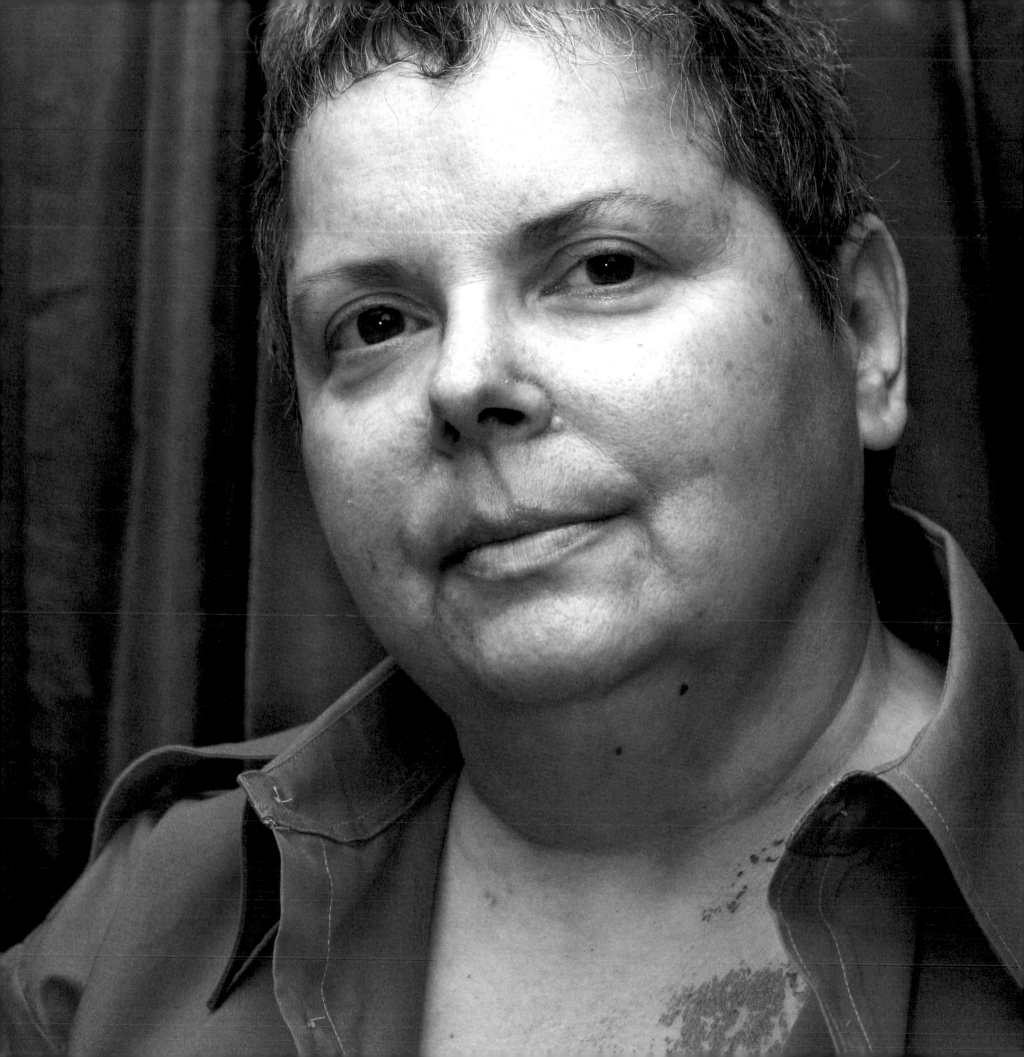

Russ

CBC broadcaster Russ
Germain stopped smoking
in 1984, after his father
died of prostate cancer.
Twenty-two years later,
however, Russ was diagnosed
with late-stage lung cancer.
In 2008 he said, "I am alive
because of new drugs,
excellent medical care, and
the love of my wife, family,
and friends. Each day is
a gift." Sadly, Russ died in
February 2009.

Photographer
Andrew Stawicki
Toronto

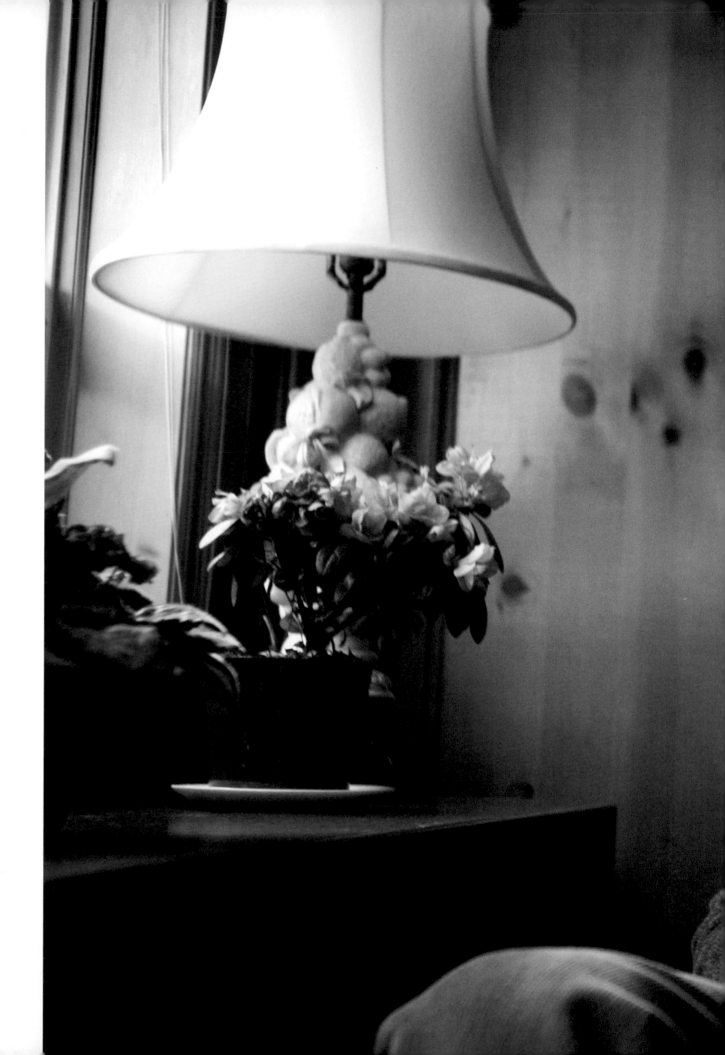

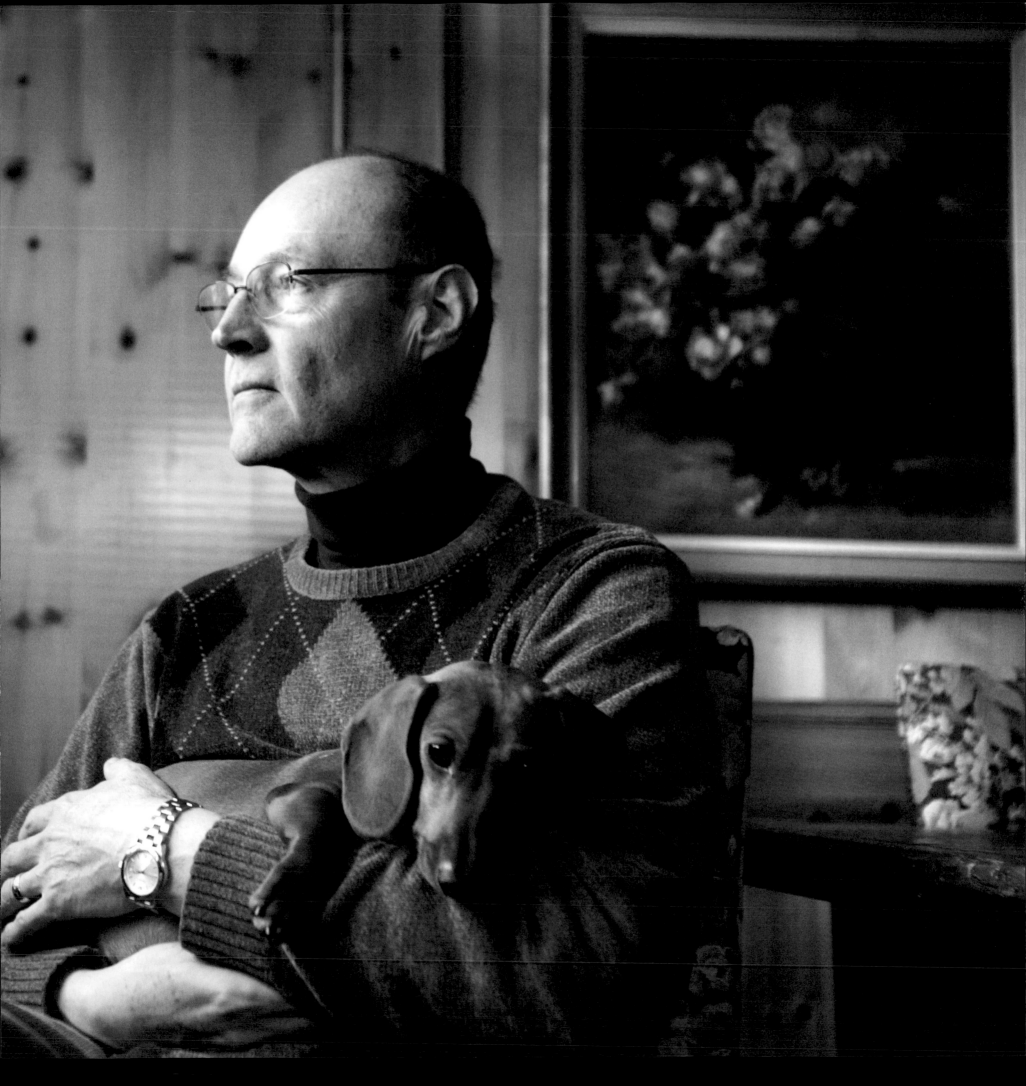

Gladys and Lalie

Twins share good and bad.
Gladys and Lalie both
battled breast cancer in
1990. Fortunately, they also
shared their 90th birthday
celebrations, in December
2007, cancer-free.

Photographer
Zuzana Capar
Toronto

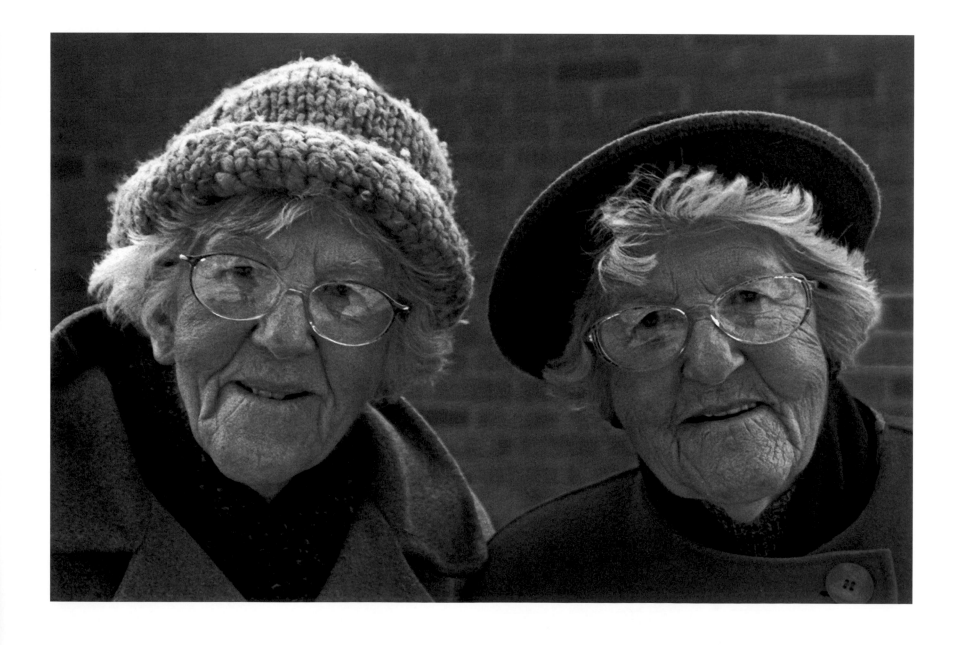

"I told the doctors, do whatever you

have to do. Take me to the very edge of death

and then pull me back."

Barbara Gadacz

Delia and Natalie

Delia and Natalie share more than a sisterly bond. Both have suffered from cancer and thrived on each other's strength, courage, optimism, and determination. Sadly, Natalie lost her battle with the disease in March 2008.

Photographer
Tobi Asmoucha
Toronto

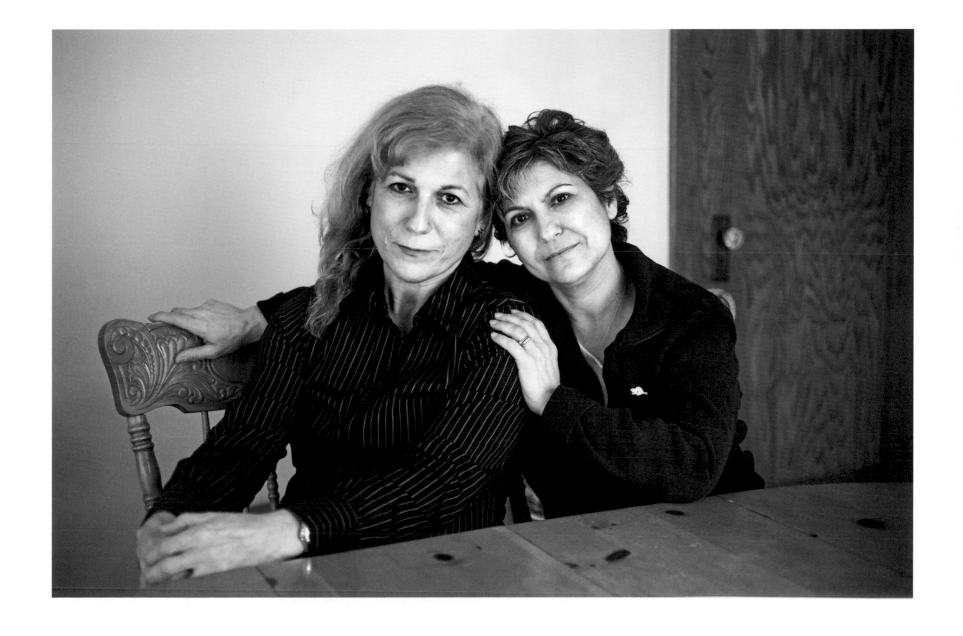

Warren

Warren Beck's mother, Judy, was undergoing breast cancer treatments at the time of this photo. She lives a two-hour drive away so he talks to her daily on the phone. She is a multiple cancer survivor.

Photographer
Lydia Charak
Toronto

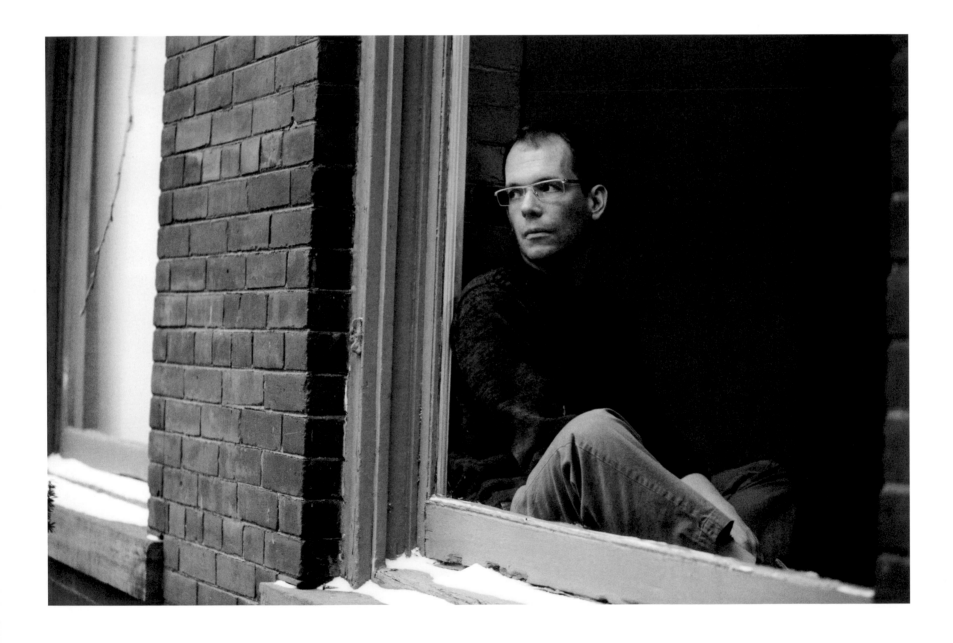

Ron

Ron Anger, husband of photographer Ellen, is a survivor of prostate cancer. The couple still has to take a deep breath before every yearly checkup, but so far he has always been given the all-clear. Ellen says, "Things aren't perfect, but he is still breathing and life is good."

Photographer
Ellen Anger
Toronto

Robert

The photographer's friend, Robert Lazariuk, at the Gilda's Club Gala, December 2005. Bryan Adams performed that evening and Gilda's Club staff arranged for Robert to meet him backstage. Five days later, after battling colon cancer for some time, Robert passed away at home. This was the last time he went out.

Photographer
Teri Henderson
Toronto

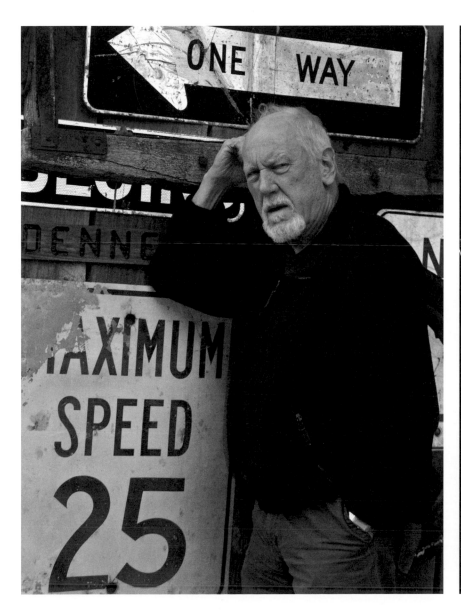

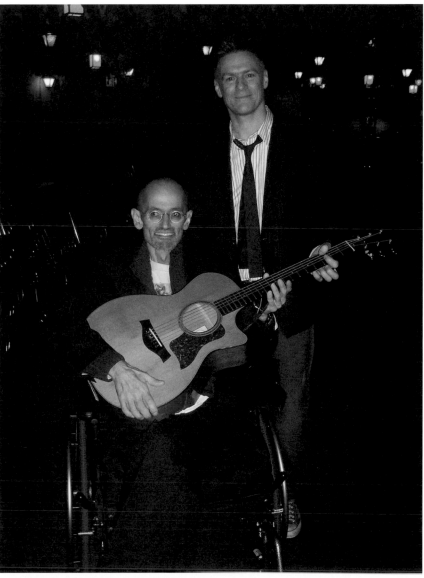

Lilah

In April 2004, doctors found a tumour the size of a golf ball in eight-pound newborn Lilah. Diagnosed with neuroblastoma, Lilah underwent numerous surgeries and chemotherapy over a six-month period. Lilah's Fund, founded by her parents to finance research into childhood cancers, has raised $300,000 so far. Lilah is now cancer-free.

Photographer
Laura Bombier
Toronto

Siva

Siva Gnanaratnam was diagnosed with a gastrointestinal stromal tumour. "Hope, courage, attitude, God, focusing on light not darkness, and family and friends have kept me alive for 14 years," she says, "along with surgery, radiation, and an experimental colon cancer drug called Gleevec."

Photographer
Irene Borins Ash
Toronto

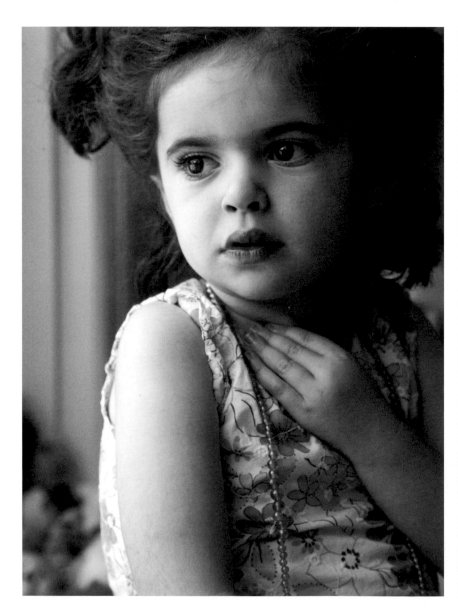

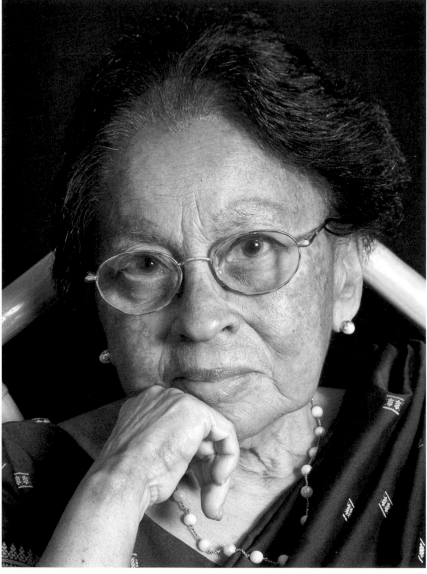

Mariellen

After being diagnosed with stage 4 colon cancer in 1999, Mariellen Black became a tireless campaigner to increase awareness about the need for screening. After listening to Mariellen, several friends went for colonoscopies, of whom three discovered they had early stage colon cancer. Today they feel they owe their lives to Mariellen. Screening might have saved Mariellen's life, had it been in place 10 years earlier.

Photographer
Andrew Stawicki
Toronto

Libby

Libby Znaimer, a breast cancer survivor, poses in Toronto, Ontario, May 2007. This photo, showing the scar over Libby's left breast, was taken within a year of her treatment. Libby then battled with pancreatic cancer and wrote a book about her experiences: *In Cancer Land*.

Photographer
Brent Foster
Toronto

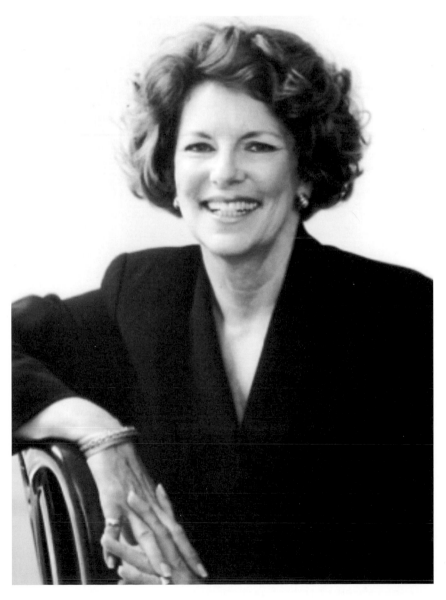

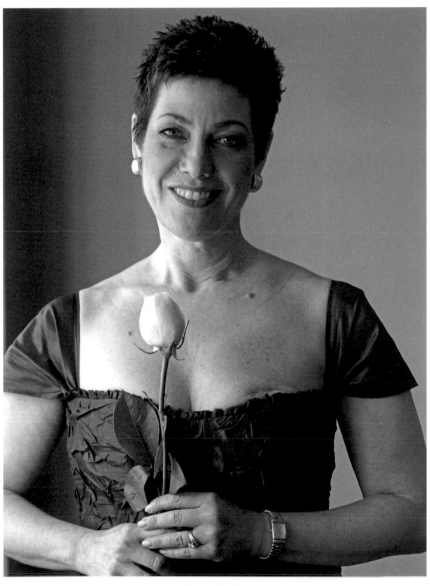

Photographer
Jeff Harris
Toronto

Jeff

Professional photographer Jeff Harris took this self-portrait, diving headfirst into a cold lake, two days after being diagnosed with neurofibrosarcoma in late 2008. "I've always enjoyed diving into water," says Jeff, "and I felt it was a neat metaphor for what I had to do."

Jeff had started a project on January 1, 1999, for which he began taking a self-portrait every day. "I wanted to make the most of every day and do something different," he says. He continues taking photos every day and posts them all on his website, www.jeffharris.org.

"With this particular photo I wanted to do something courageous," says Jeff. "I was conscious that I was about to jump into a crappy, uncomfortable experience. I said to myself, 'I will do it, it will be over soon, and I will feel better for it.'"

Jeff's diagnosis was a long time in coming. He first began experiencing back pain and shooting pains down his leg in July 2007, but due to the nature of the cancer, it took 16 months to be diagnosed. "It was a soft tissue tumour, so it can hide in there really well," explains Jeff. "The good news was that meant it was a slow-growing tumour."

An MRI revealed that the tumour was on his sciatic nerve, thus the shooting pains, and a biopsy revealed that the cancer was growing through his pelvis, attaching itself to his tailbone and half of his sacrum. Before surgery, Jeff went through five weeks of radiation to create larger margins around the tumour to make for an easier surgery.

For the 11-hour, highly invasive surgery, Jeff lay on his side while an orthopedic surgeon worked on his back and a gastroenterology surgeon worked on his front. The surgery was successful in removing the tumour but left Jeff's body in disrepair. Part of his pelvis was removed, which caused his right leg to rise up into his pelvis and become considerably shorter. His left leg became permanently paralyzed from the knee down; it has since withered and the muscles have atrophied.

None of this deterred Jeff from embracing the healing process. Eighteen months after surgery he was taking physiotherapy twice a week, attending yoga classes, and having still-healing wounds attended to daily by a nurse. "The cancer was removed fairly quickly, but I now have a lifetime of side effects to deal with."

The nature of Jeff's daily photos also changed. "I now take photos in which I don't seem so much like a cancer patient with paralysis—like standing over a river on a fallen tree, without my crutches. Up to a point I have been deprived of my ability to have adventure. In taking these kinds of photos, I make a conscious effort to have adventures regardless."

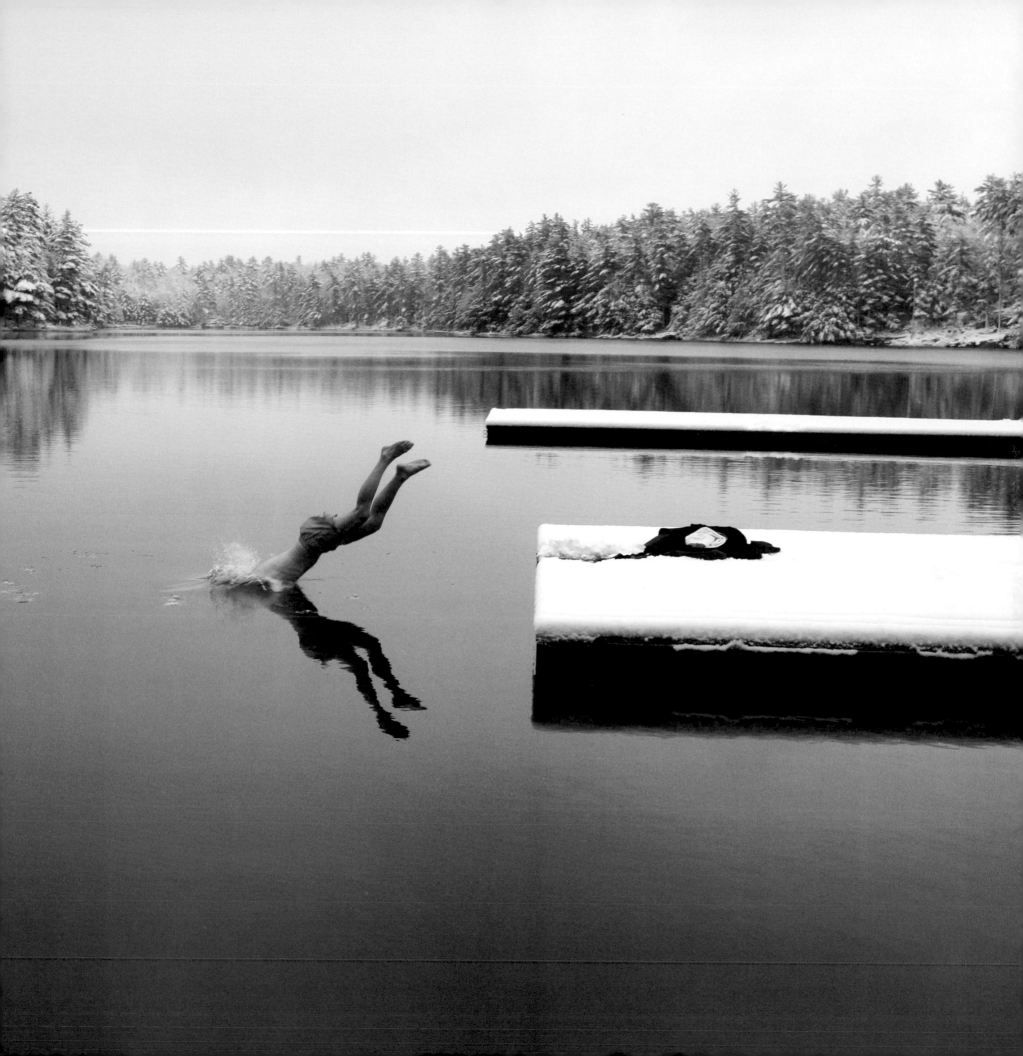

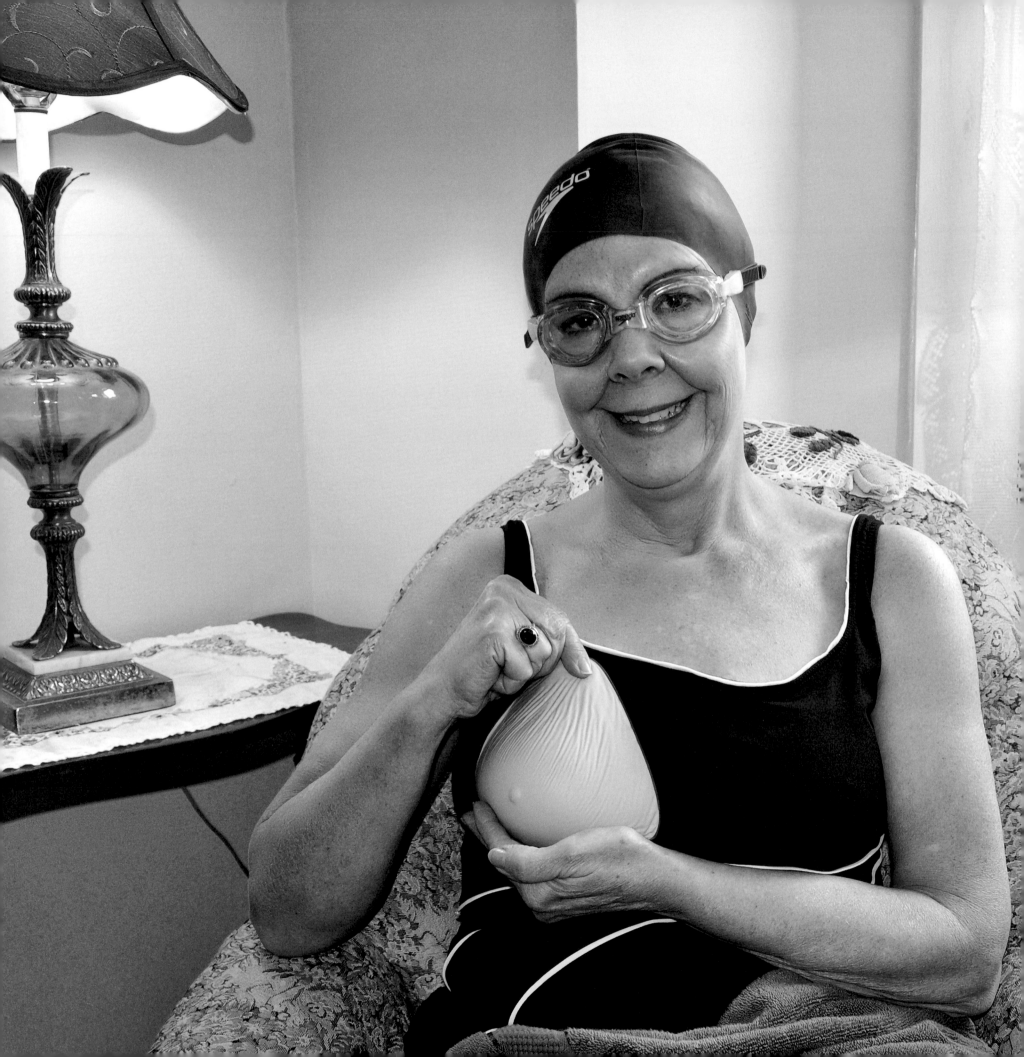

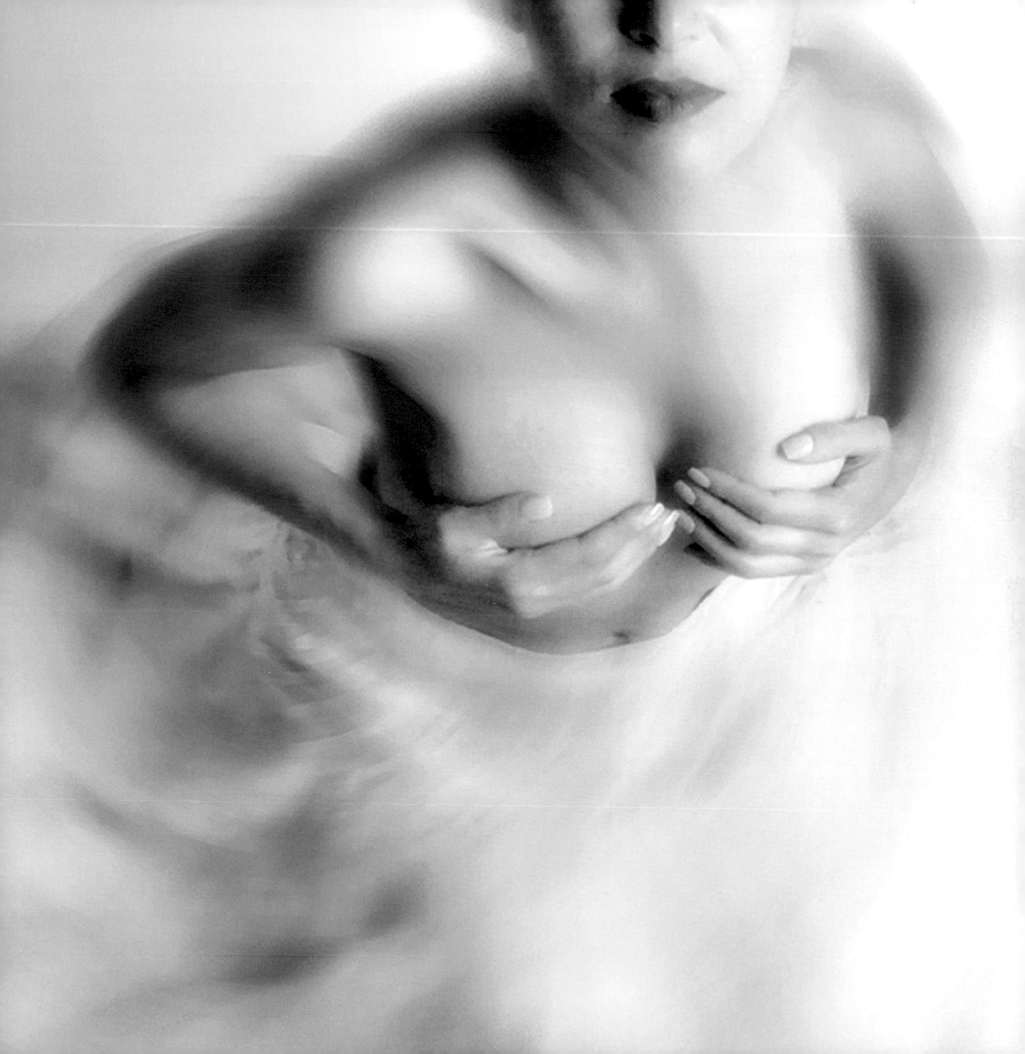

Previous left

Jane

Jane, a keen swimmer, had pre-cancerous cells discovered in her right breast two years ago. After the resection of the breast, Jane chose to use a prosthesis, which she has named Fred, rather than have reconstructive surgery. She is seen holding Fred in an appropriate position to substitute for the original breast. Jane is now fine and has resumed swimming.

Photographer
Mary Perdue
Toronto

Previous right

Margarida

Margarida was diagnosed with cancer at the age of 27. She has survived and thrived, proving that, even after a mastectomy, you can still be 100 per cent woman. "Live life to the fullest," she says. "The race is long and in the end it's only with yourself."

Photographer
Michele Taras
Toronto

Carol

Carol Crealock, a university professor, was diagnosed with oligodendroglioma (a type of brain tumour) at the age of 47. After surgery and treatment, she found accessing her vocabulary to be difficult. Nevertheless, she continued to teach, research, and publish for 11 more years. She died of advanced stomach cancer in 2006, aged 65.

Photographer
Molly Crealock
Toronto

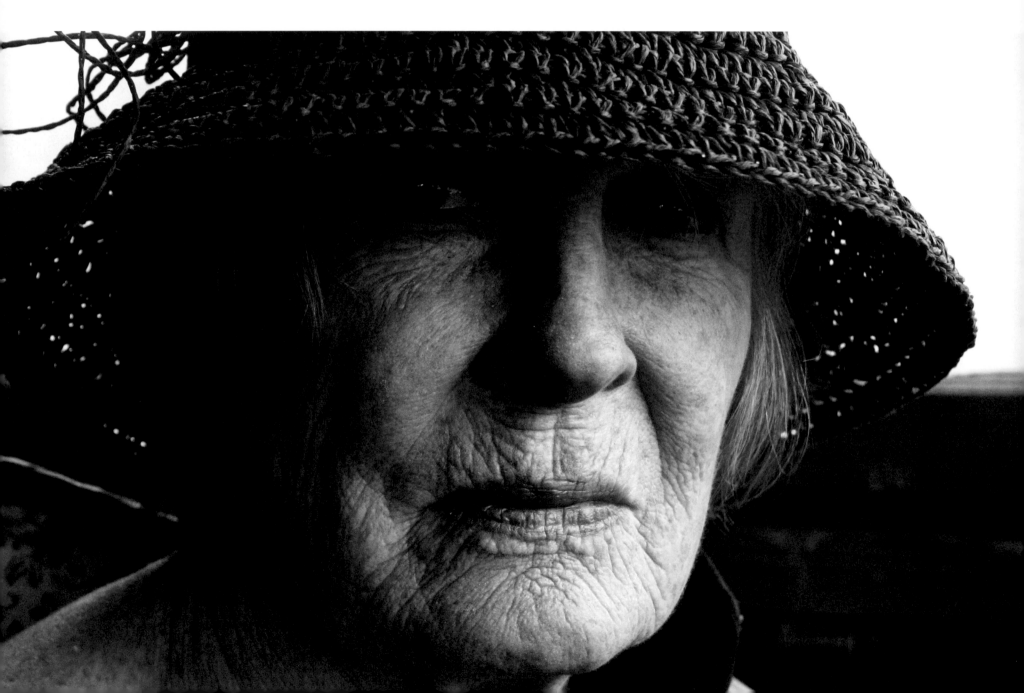

June

June Callwood, journalist, author, social activist, and good friend of PhotoSensitive, fought cancer for several years before succumbing to the disease in 2007. She encouraged PhotoSensitive to produce *Cancer Connections*, saying, "It's high time someone did something really inspired."

Photographer
V. Tony Hauser
Toronto

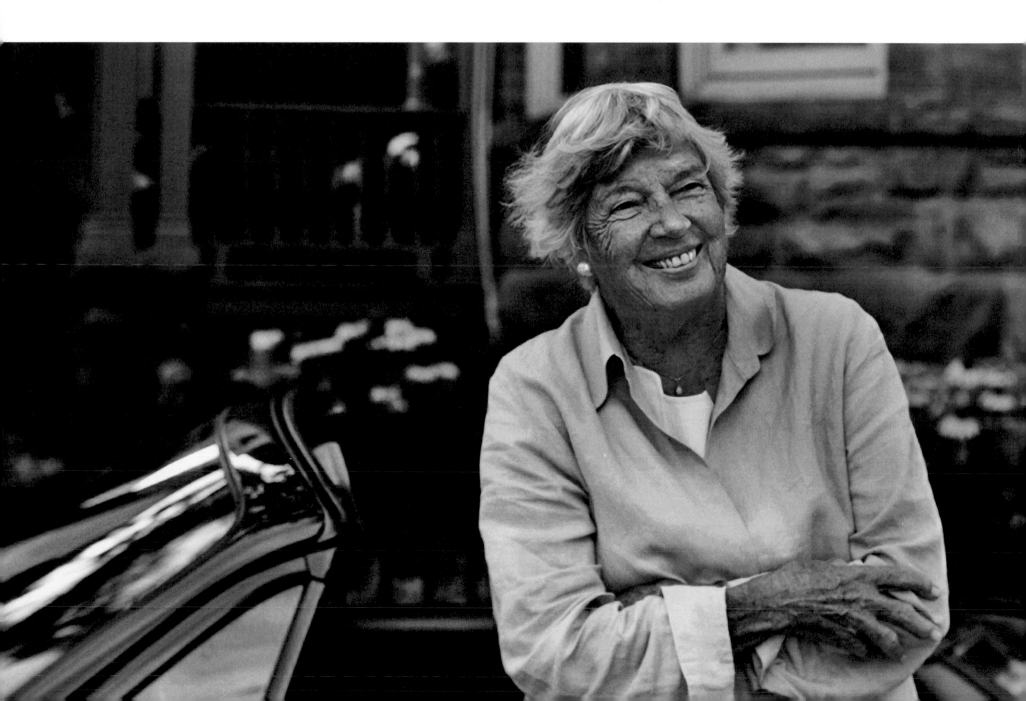

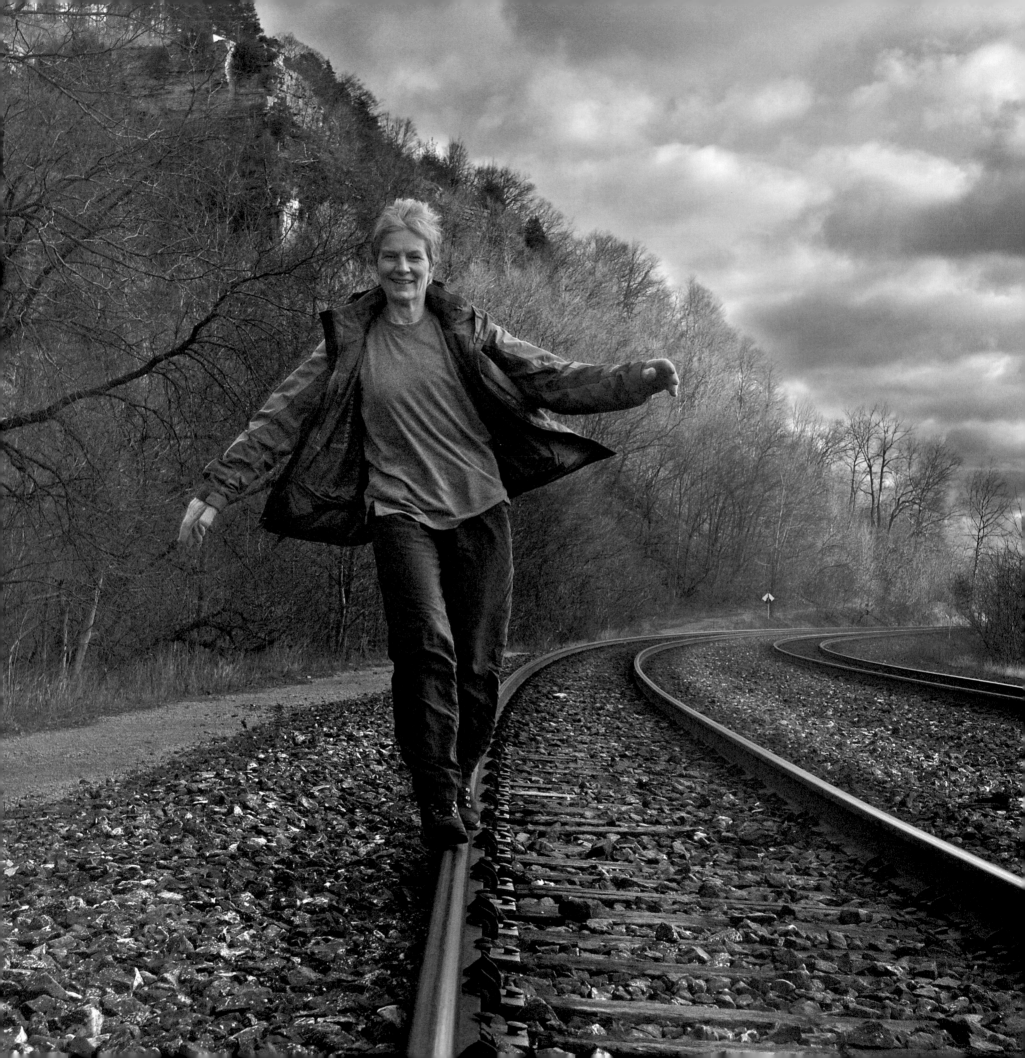

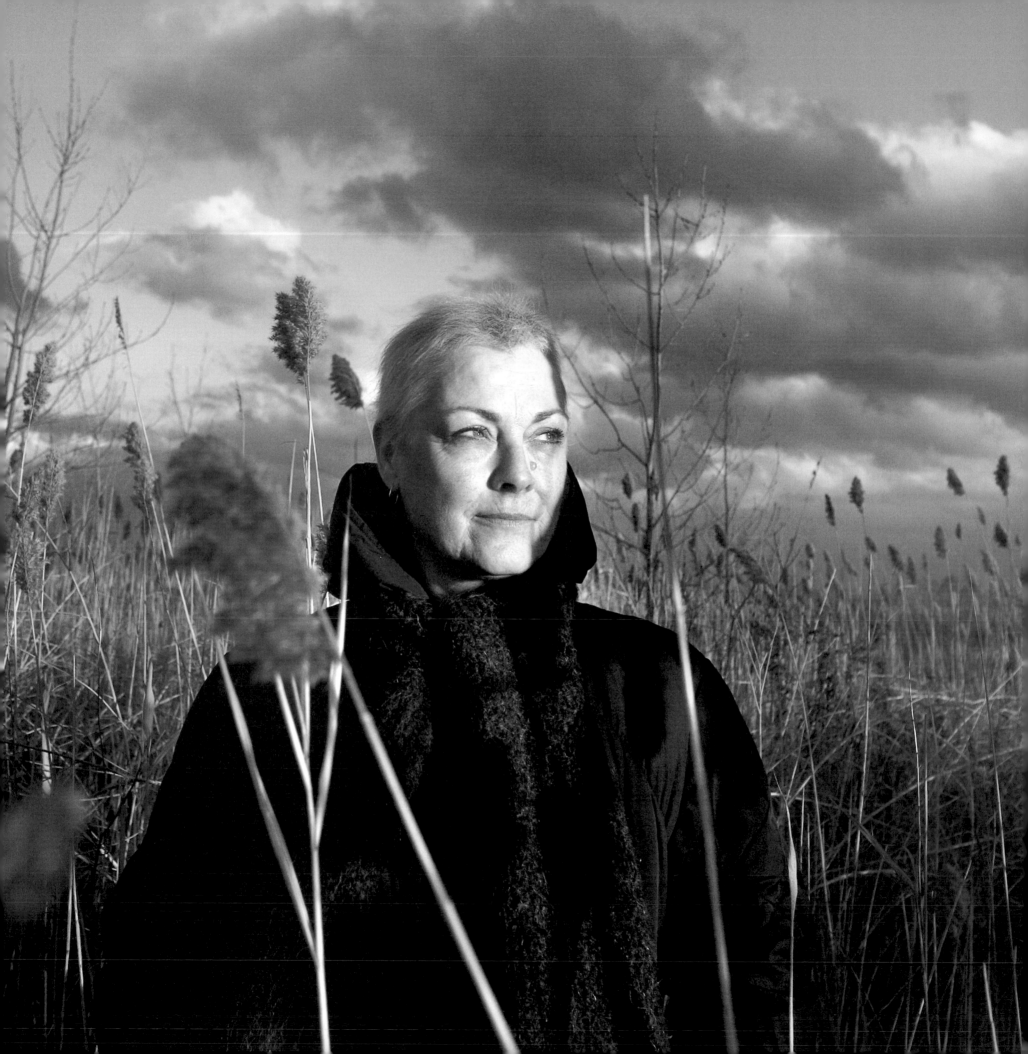

Previous left

Jane

Jane is one of the lucky
ones: This quilt maker
survived breast cancer in
1994. Since then, she
has had a heightened
appreciation of all aspects
of life.

Photographer
Tessa Buchan
Toronto

Previous right

Anne

Anne Edwards was diag-
nosed with ovarian cancer
in 2006; she was told that
the cancer had spread
beyond her ovaries. Anne
underwent surgery and
received chemotherapy at
Sunnybrook Cancer Centre
in Toronto, Ontario.
In August 2007 she was
told that she was in
remission.

Photographer
Chris Young
Toronto

Naomi and Sara

Naomi Engel (left) had
just finished her chemotherapy for breast cancer
as her friend Sara Cotton
was beginning hers for
lymphoma. "It was great to
have someone to talk to who
had already been through
chemotherapy," says Sara.
"It was very reassuring."
Both are now cancer-free.

Photographer
Pixie Shaw
Toronto

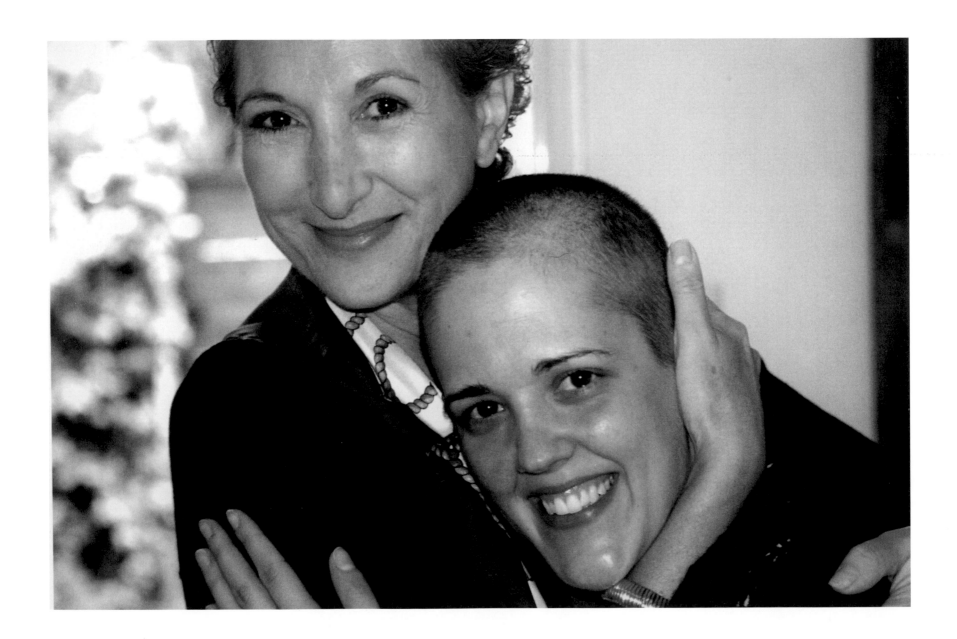

Juliana and Zelia

Juliana, now in stage 4 of terminal cancer, lies with her daughter Zelia, who is her primary caregiver.

Photographer
Steve Stober
Toronto

Alex and Tracey

Alex Lawson, 55, was diagnosed with cancer of the liver in 2006 and put on a waiting list for a donor. But his condition deteriorated so quickly that his sister Tracey Allan, 43, a mother of two, offered to donate part of her liver. The two operations went well, and both brother and sister are in good health.

Photographer
Dick Loek
Toronto

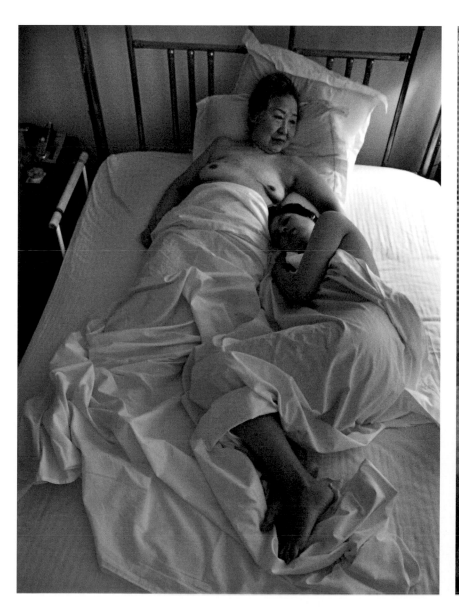

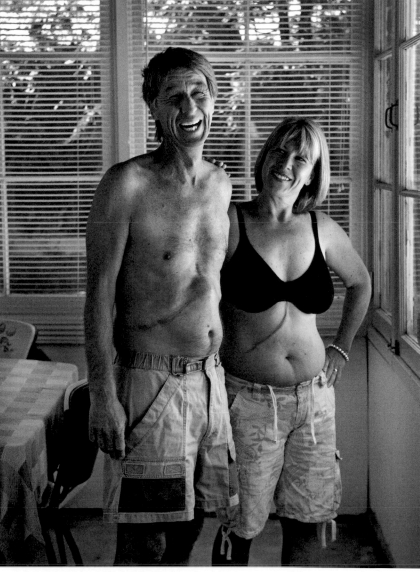

Opposite

Rachel

At the age of four, Rachel was diagnosed with choroidal melanoma and had to have an eye removed. In spite of this, she is a happy six-year-old who likes to read, skate, and help others coping with eye cancer with her book, *I Can … Eye Can*.

Photographer
Stan Behal
Toronto

Manon

Manon Zigelstein was three when she was diagnosed with lymphoblastic leukemia in 2006. Between then and April 2008, when this photo was taken, she lost her hair twice to chemotherapy. Halfway through her treatment, she dreamt that the tooth fairy was going to make her well.

Photographer
Anka Czudec
Toronto

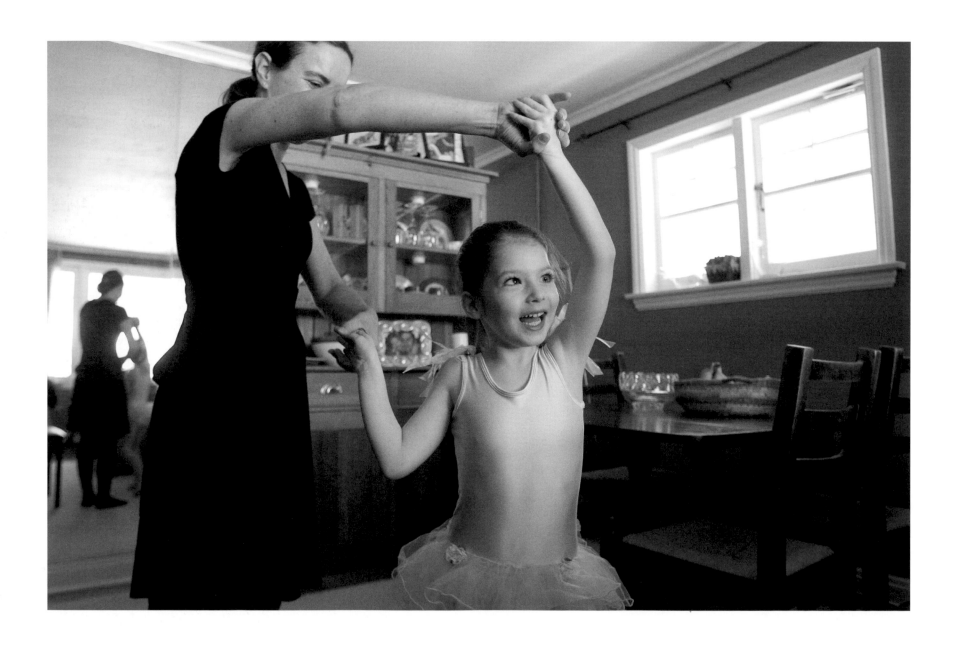

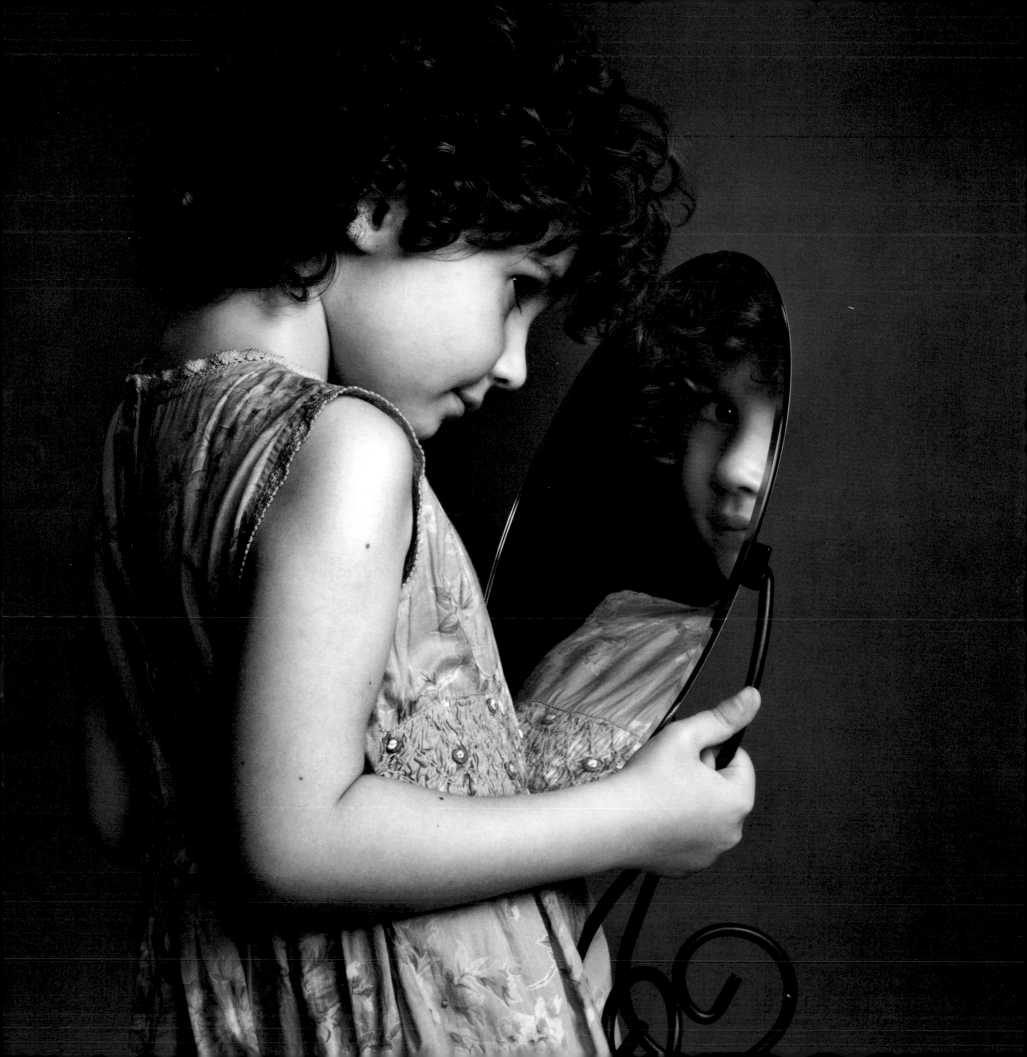

Bruce

Bruce Horak lost his right eye to retinoblastoma and cancer claimed the life of his father. He now personifies the disease in a one-man show—"This is Cancer: Live"—with a mandate of healing through humour. He says, "I don't think there's a more absurd way to deal with cancer than to play cancer."

Photographer
Jill Kitchener
Toronto

Dreas

Dreas Reyneke, now in his mid-70s, has been an internationally renowned Pilates teacher for decades. He is now suffering from follicular lymphoma, a common type of non-Hodgkin's lymphoma.

Photographer
Yuri Dojc
Toronto

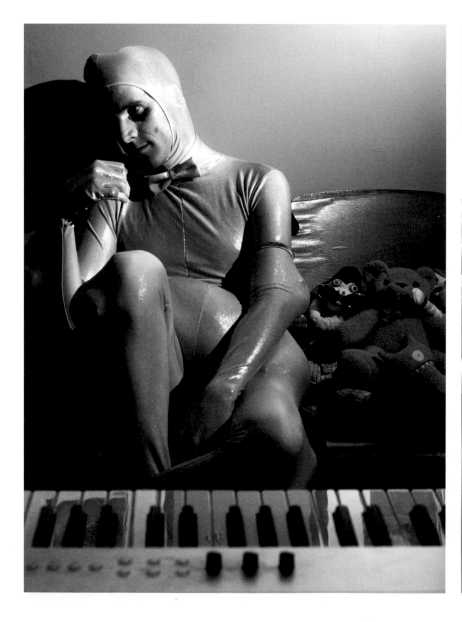

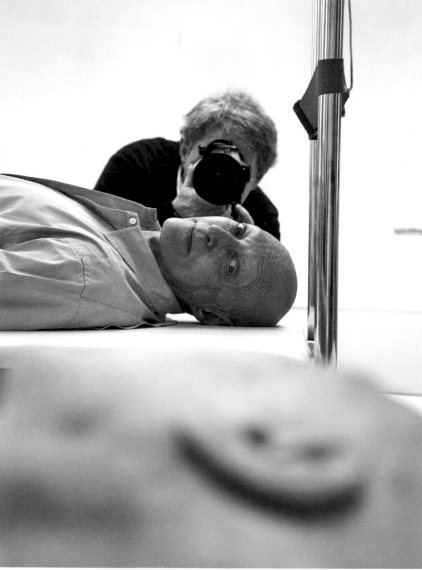

"I don't think there's a more absurd way to

deal with cancer than to play cancer."

Bruce Horak

Sharon

Sharon Hampson, of the
musical trio Sharon,
Lois & Bram, is a mother
of two, three-time breast
cancer survivor, and
co-founder of Willow Breast
Cancer Support Canada,
which provides information
to those living with the
disease. "Doing something
that helps others deal
with this hardship is a real
gift to me," she says.

Photographer
Peter Bregg
Toronto

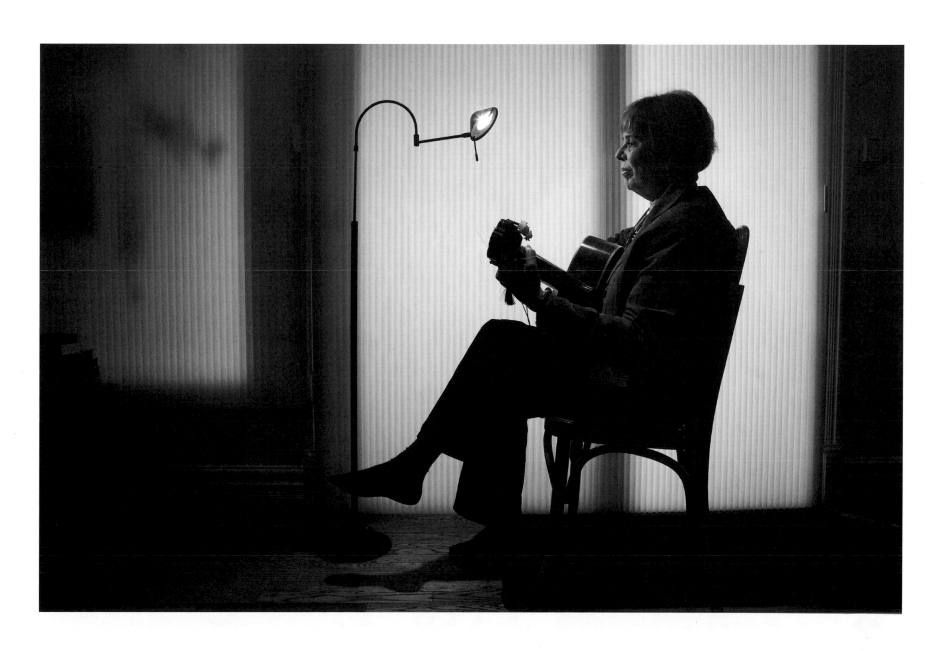

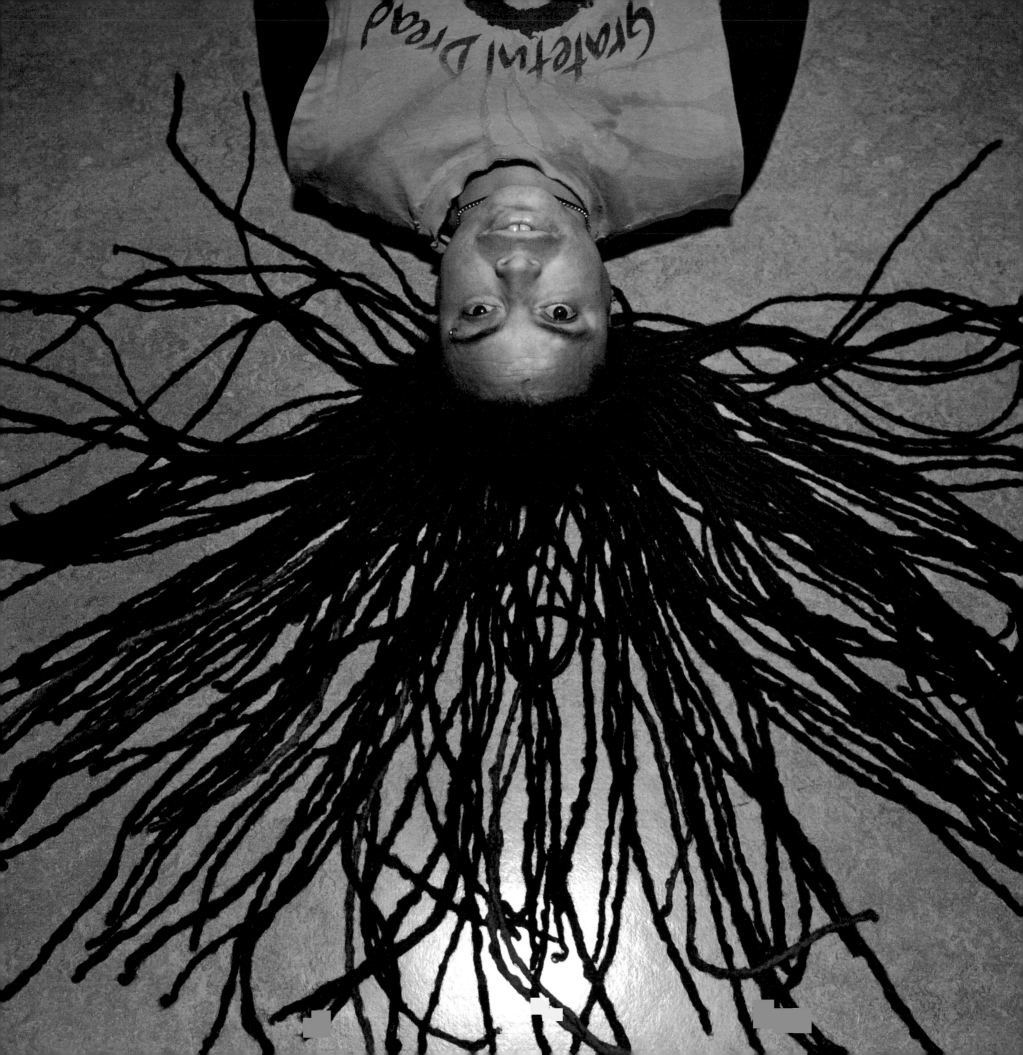

Opposite

Lorelei

At the age of three, a
tumour was discovered
in Lorelei King's left eye;
she was diagnosed with
retinoblastoma and surgeons
removed the eye. Since
then Lorelei has made a full
recovery and gone on
to become an active and
inspirational leader in
her community.

Photographer
Kevin Van Paassen
Toronto

Keith

After being diagnosed
with colon cancer,
Keith took the first of
his daily self-portraits. He
says, "I had to get used to
the 'subject,' and ignore
the 'me.' I could stop
worrying about my
cancer, because I would
be too busy in pursuit
of photos of Keith."

Photographer
Keith Branscombe
Toronto

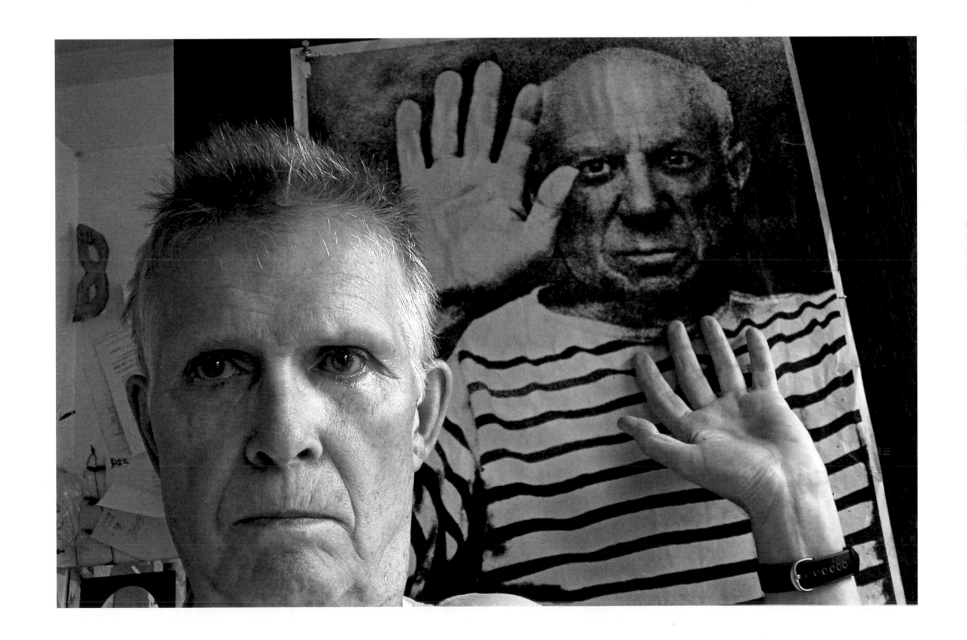

Row 1: Adriana Burigana, Toronto; Ali Thompson, Toronto; Ania Kohinski, Toronto; Arline Malakian (4–5), Toronto; Ashley Hutcheson, Toronto; Barbara Cassidy, Toronto; Barbara Stoneham, Toronto

Row 2: Barry Shainbaum, Toronto; Benjamin Rondell (2–5), Toronto, Brenda Howard, Toronto; Brennan O'Connor, Toronto; Bryonie Wise, Toronto

Row 3: C. Taeuschel (1–2), Toronto; Carol Mark, Toronto; Cheol Joon Baek, Toronto; Chris Ablett, Toronto; Chris McCallan, Toronto; Chris Young, Toronto; Daniel Stolfi,Toronto

Row 4: Daniel Stolfi (1–2), Toronto; Daria Perevezentsev (3–7), Toronto; David Christen, Toronto

Row 5: David Christen, Toronto; David Hou, Toronto; Dean Oros, Toronto; Deanna Bickford, Toronto; Deborah Martin, Toronto; Dodie McNally (6–8), Toronto

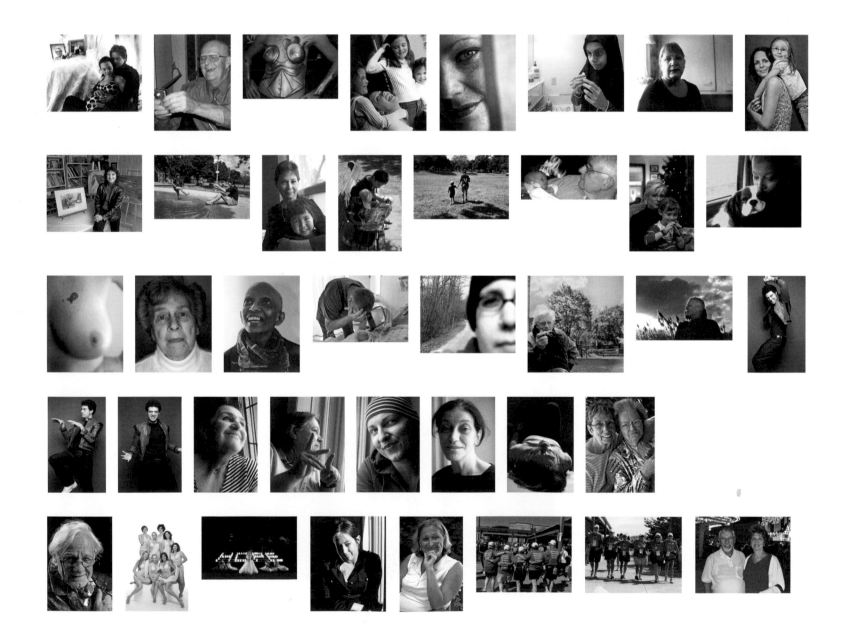

Row 1: Eileen Herbert, Toronto; Ellen Anger (2–3), Toronto; Ethan Mitchell, Toronto; Giulio Muratori, Toronto; Grace Van Berkum (6–8), Toronto

Row 2: Graig Abel, Toronto; Heather Babin (2–3), Toronto; Heidi Ricafort, Toronto; Hugh Wesley (5–8), Toronto

Row 3: Jackie Osmond Patrick (1–4), Toronto; Janice Hardacre, Toronto; Jasmine Bakalarz, Toronto; Jeff Harris (7–8), Toronto

Row 4: Jeff Harris (1–6), Toronto; Jill Kitchener (7–8), Toronto

Row 5: Jim Rankin, Toronto; Joel Walker, Toronto; Jon Vopni (3–4), Toronto; Jonathan Fox, Toronto; Josefina Nadurata, Toronto; Keith Branscombe (7–8), Toronto

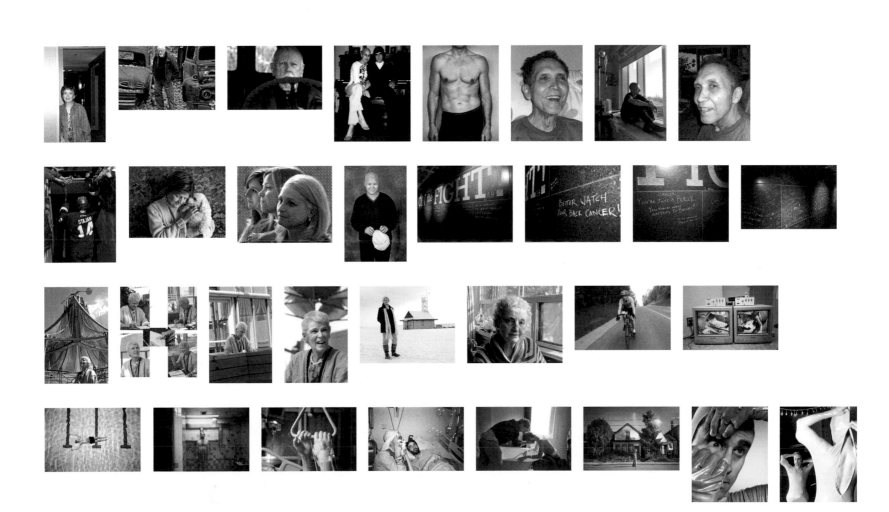

Row 1: Keith Branscombe, Toronto; Kelly Gauthier (2–8), Toronto

Row 2: Kelly Gauthier, Toronto; Kevin Lam, Toronto; Kiana Hayeri-Joabi, Toronto; Kimberly Shek (4–6), Toronto;
Kim Vose Jones (7–8), Toronto

Row 3: Kristen Joy Watts, Toronto; Larry Frank, Toronto; Larry Zeligson, Toronto; Laura Bombier, Toronto; Lawrence Salza, Toronto;
Leehe Lev, Toronto; Linda Cresswell, Rene Belzile, & Jett Tano (7–8),Toronto

Row 4: Linda Cresswell, Rene Belzile, & Jett Tano, Toronto; Lino Torrado, Toronto; Margaret Whewall, Toronto;
Mark Manchester, Toronto; Michele Clarke, Toronto; Michelle Yee, Toronto; Nancy Paiva, Toronto; Nandini Saxena, Toronto

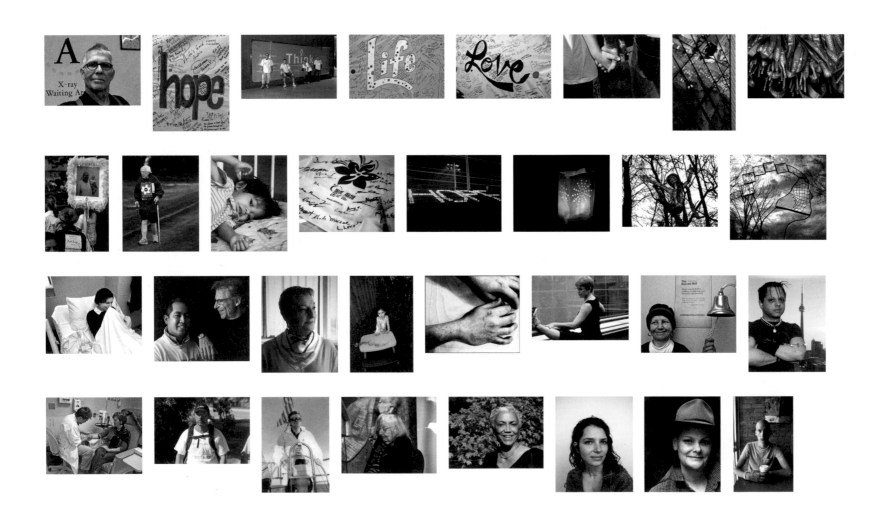

Row 1: Ozren Stambuk, Toronto; Paul Sergeant, Toronto; Petra King, Toronto; Robin Rowland, Toronto; Robyn Smale, Toronto; Ron Jocsak, Toronto; Sabu Qureshi, Toronto; Sachi Maruyama, Toronto

Row 2: Sairaa Astaria Thornton, Toronto; Salina Kassam, Toronto; Sally Cumming, Toronto; Samantha Young, Toronto; Sarah Tothill, Toronto; Sharon Bedard, Toronto; Sharon Reynolds, Toronto; Stan Behal, Toronto

Row 3: Talia Baldor, Toronto; Tanya Workman, Toronto; Taylor Zhou, Toronto; Ted Bridgewater, Toronto; Thereza Suzuki (5–7), Toronto

Row 4: Thereza Suzuki (1–2), Toronto; Wendy Rombough, Toronto

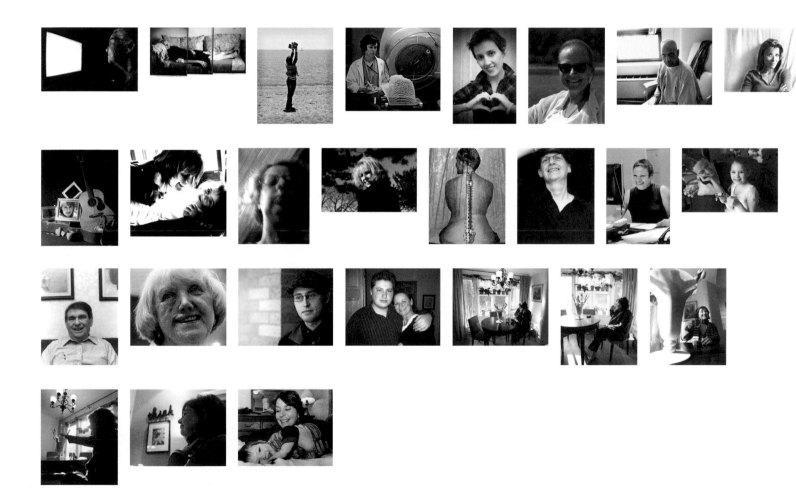

Quebec

"Cancer challenged me to live my life as I want and to focus on what's uniquely important to me."

Tiana Cornelius

Photographer
Elizabeth Knox
Montreal

Tiana

When she was only 17, Tiana Cornelius noticed a bump on the right side of her face. "I immediately knew that something was really wrong," she recalls. "Everyone was saying I was too young for it to be anything serious. My doctor said it was an inner ear infection and gave me antibiotics."

When the bump continued to grow, Tiana had a small needle biopsy, which proved inconclusive. Two weeks later, after a major surgical biopsy, she was told that she might have incurable cancer. It took another two weeks before she got the correct diagnosis: she had alveolar rhabdomyosarcoma. She was relieved to learn that it was treatable and that she had an 80 per cent chance of recovery.

"It was a completely overwhelming and scary time," says Tiana. "I had just turned 18 and thought that I was going to die. You shouldn't have to deal with your own mortality when your life is just beginning to take shape."

Tiana's tumour was exceptionally aggressive, having grown from the size of a pea in September to eight centimetres in diameter by December. The treatment had to be equally aggressive and Tiana began a 10-month course of chemotherapy and radiation, which included an experimental drug.

Tiana responded well to the chemotherapy—the cancer shrank to nothing and was undetectable after the first two months of

treatment. She has been cancer-free ever since, but the treatment was arduous. "I received excessive amounts of chemo and radiation. For three months after completing therapy I couldn't feel or move my toes. I felt weak and got sick constantly for years. It took two to three years for my body to rebuild and recover completely."

Thankfully, Tiana has had no long-term side effects from the treatment and the whole experience has proven a positive one in many respects.

"I am more resilient and less concerned about trivialities. Cancer challenged me to live my life as I want and focus on what's uniquely important to me. Life is short and can change drastically, or end, at any time. I take more risks than most people because I want to maximize every moment I have. I'm also less afraid to put myself out there—nothing is more humbling than going through chemotherapy."

For her *Cancer Connections* photo, taken by her friend Elizabeth Knox, Tiana dressed up to reflect her personal style and struck a theatrical pose. "I didn't want the photo to reflect the negativity of cancer. I'm not mired in suffering. Beating cancer made me a stronger and more beautiful person."

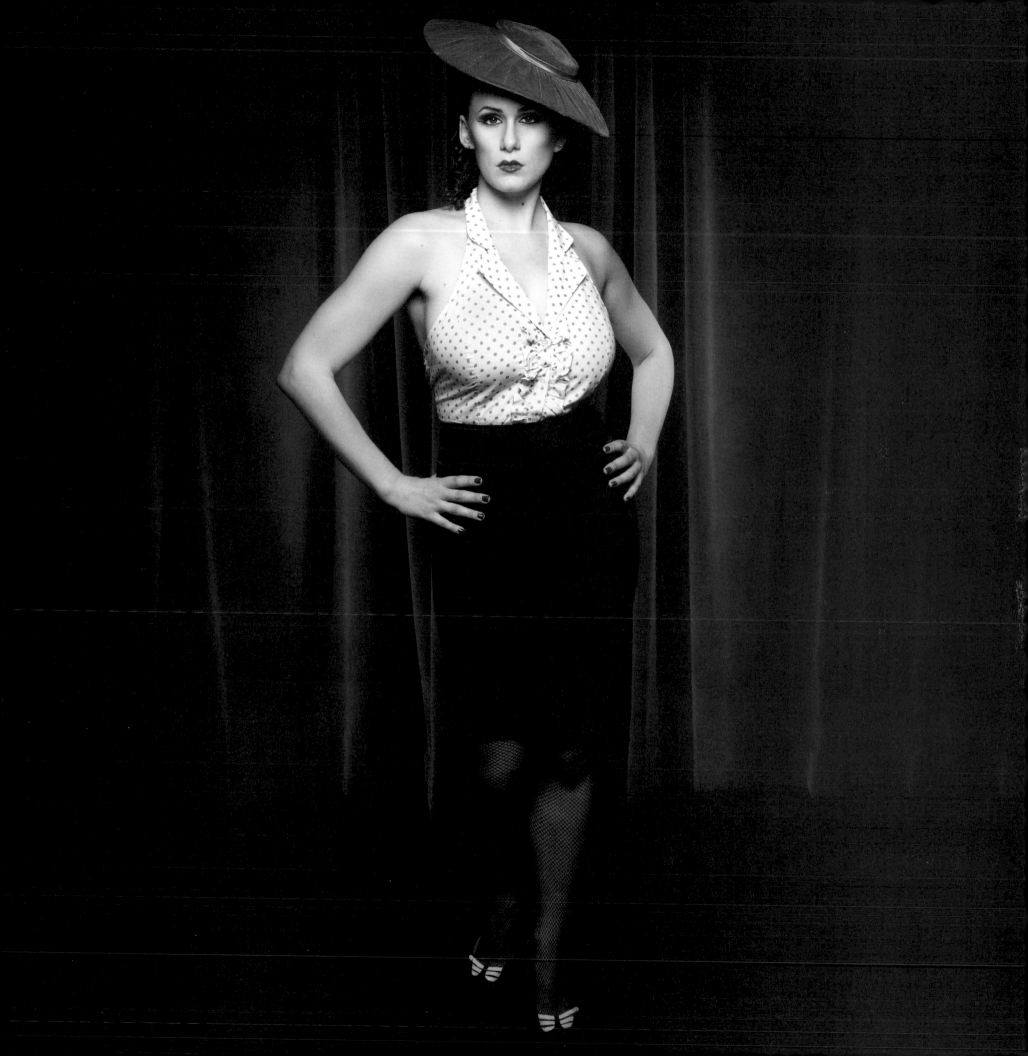

for being there
ach and every day
ove Love Love Lo
sion Passion Pass
mpassion Compas

Previous

Anna and David

When a woman loses one or both breasts, is she less feminine? After losing her breasts to cancer six years ago, Anna has increasingly tapped into her inner sensual powers. Her husband, David, lost his first wife to cancer; four years after marrying David, Anna was diagnosed with breast cancer.

Photographer
Hera Bell
Mont St-Hilaire

Louise and Jay

Jay with his mother, Louise, who was diagnosed with a rare and aggressive cancer when Jay was 20. Given a 50 per cent survival chance, Louise decided that death was not an option, that her husband and sons needed her. Jay was with his mother for every step of her treatment, confident that she would overcome the disease. Louise is now in remission.

Photographer
Yves Choquette
Montreal

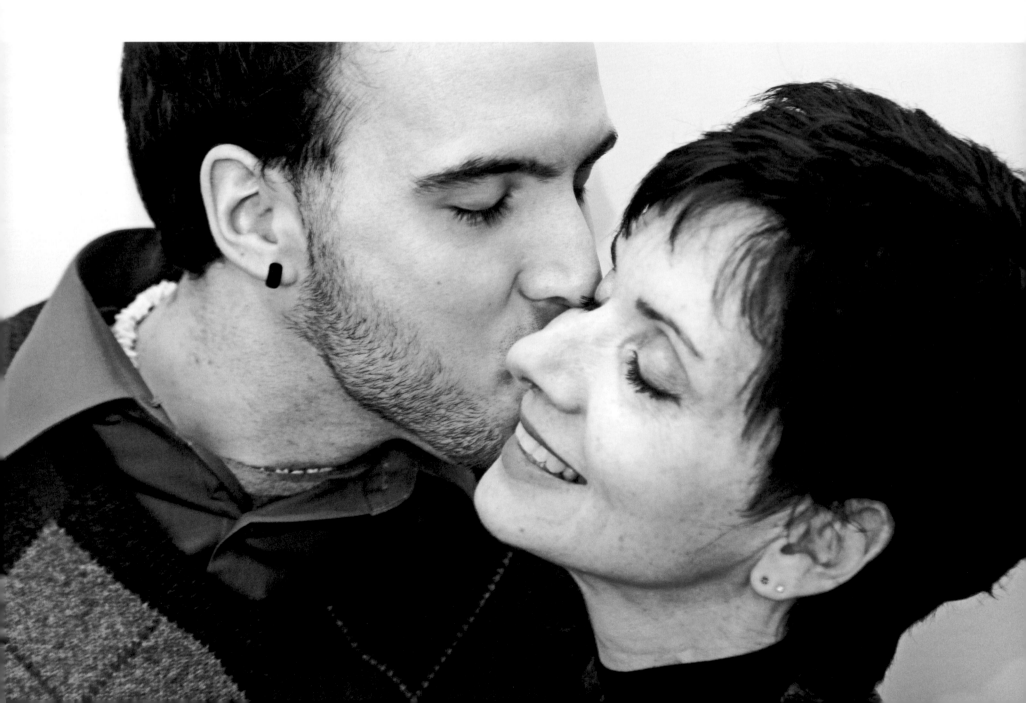

Isabelle and Ansha

Isabelle Massé, 36, with her daughter Ansha. Isabelle is a carrier of the potentially breast cancer-inducing BRCA2 gene. She, her grandmother, mother, and sister have all had cancer. Isabelle says, "May God give me the strength to live to see the day when my daughter can live without suffering from this disease."

Photographer
René Rioux
Ste-Edwidge-de-Clifton

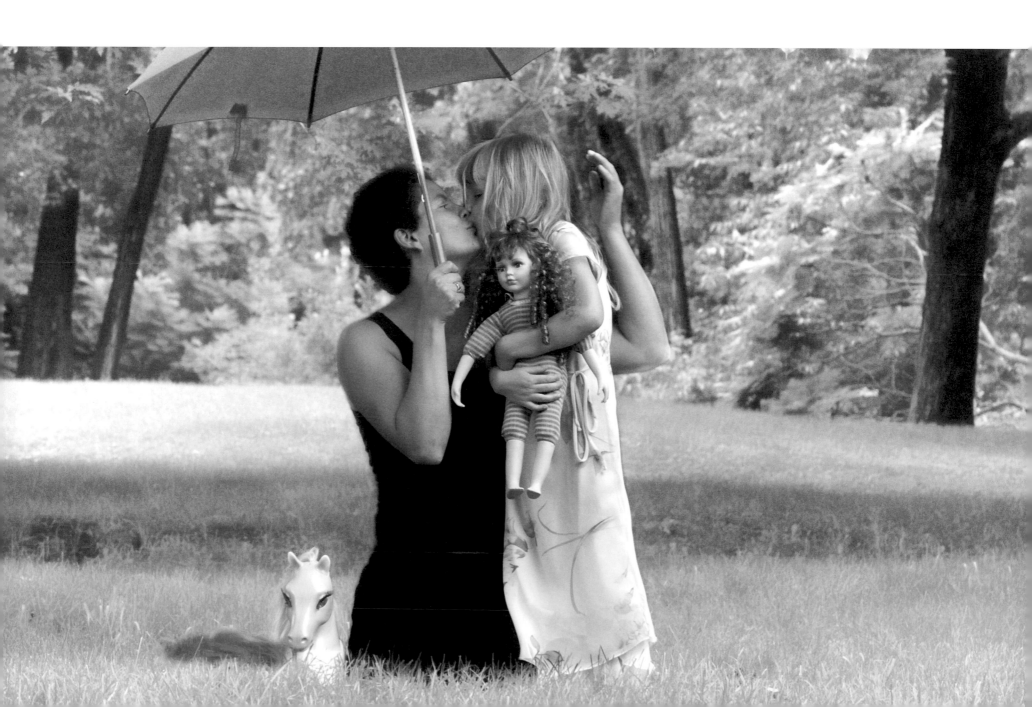

Photographer
Vicky Vriniotis
Pierrefonds

Emru

When Emru Townsend attended the *Cancer Connections* opening ceremony in Montreal in September 2008 with his wife, photographer Vicky Vriniotis, he was already 10 months into his cancer journey.

In November 2007, Emru had been feeling ill, with an insatiable thirst and a craving for only fruit. He was finally diagnosed with diabetes insipidus, a condition characterized by excessive thirst, but doctors were not sure what had caused it. Tests finally revealed that Emru had acute myelogenous leukemia.

After Emru's first of three cycles of chemotherapy, doctors told him that he would need a bone marrow transplant since he also had a secondary condition called monosomy 7. Emru's sister Tamu was not a match, so his only hope was to find a matching donor on the national and international donor registries.

An animation and technology writer and blogger, Emru decided to be proactive in his search for a donor and launched a website, healemru.com, on which he blogged about his experience and encouraged people to join the registry. "His demeanor was, 'I am going to meet this head on,'" says Vicky. "He never said, 'Why me?'"

Given his Afro-Caribbean background, Emru's chances of finding a donor were slimmer because his ethnicity was under-represented in donor registries. "We didn't just set up the website for Emru," says Vicky. "We wanted to help other cancer patients as well by encouraging people to join the registry. In the summer of 2008 an anonymous donor was found."

A combination of his ethnicity and the fact that he had both leukemia and monosomy 7 meant that doctors were not overly optimistic about Emru's hopes of recovery. "They said there was a one in seven chance that Emru would survive," says Vicky. "But they also said that he didn't have much choice but to try for the transplant."

The transplant was a success in many ways except for the important one: the leukemia didn't go into remission and Emru passed away on November 11, 2008. "I never imagined being a widow at 41," says Vicky. "We said till death us do part, but I didn't think it would be so soon."

For Vicky, her son Max and her family were essential in overcoming her loss. "Emru told his doctor that I am stronger than I think and he was right. Having both sets of grandparents actively involved in our lives, we have adjusted to not having Emru around, but in my head I can still picture him walking through the door. The important thing was that Emru did everything he could to save himself. There are no regrets."

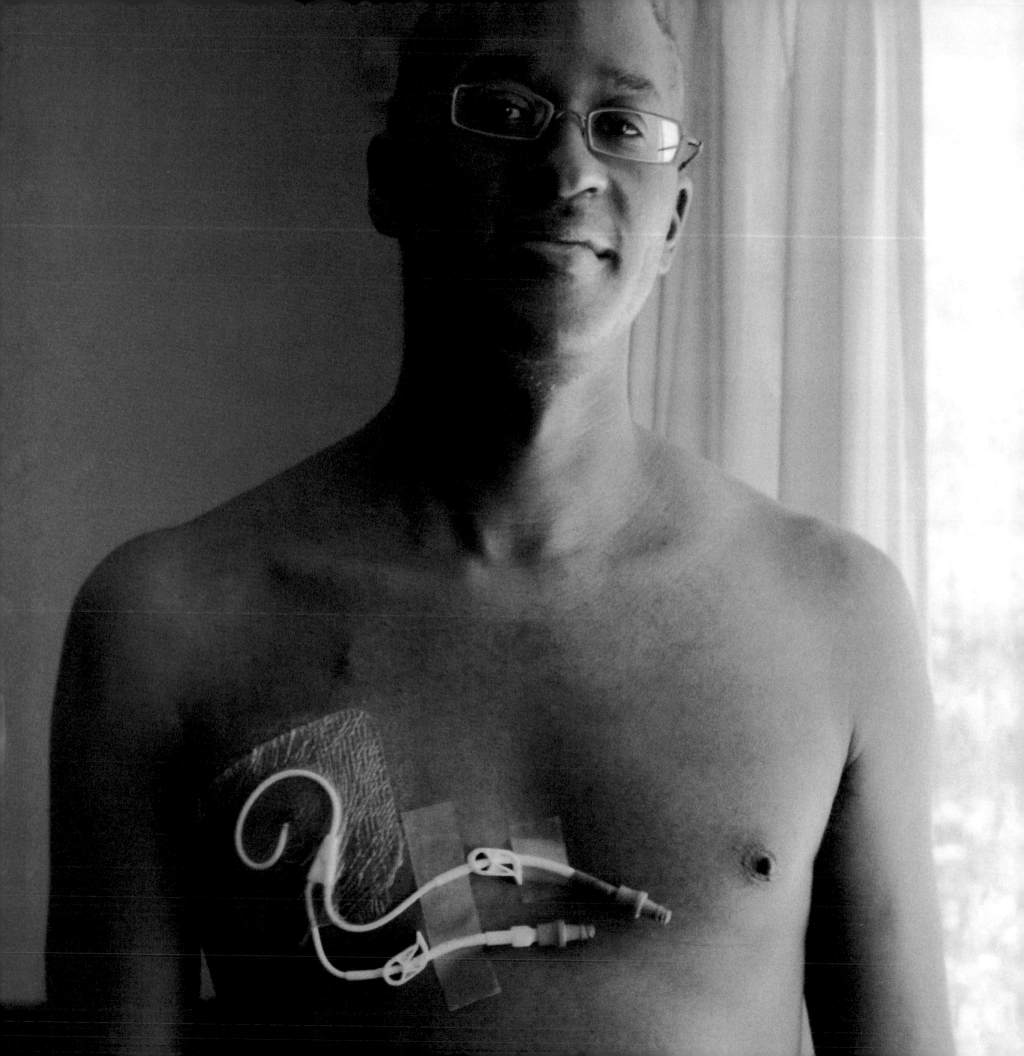

Debbie

Debbie Parkes, a colleague and friend of the photographer, the week before her second mastectomy surgery, July 2006 in Montreal.

Photographer
Phil Carpenter
St. Bruno

Suzanne

Suzanne Birtz won her battle with breast cancer, but not without scars. Luma R. Brieuc, the photographer and a henna artist, has known Suzanne for two years and says, "I created the henna butterfly to accompany her through this transformation of her body and hope it gave her wings to fly."

Photographer
Luma Rafaelle Brieuc
Montreal

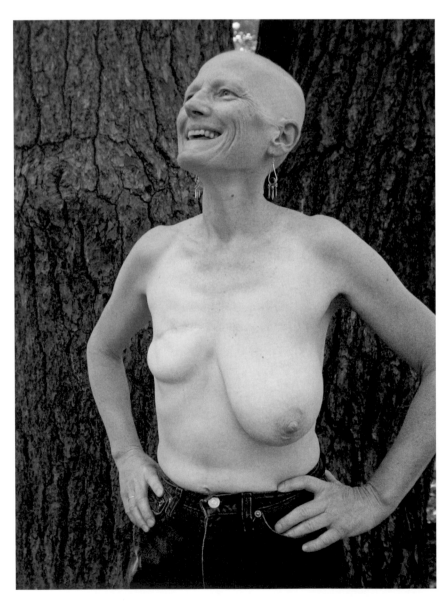

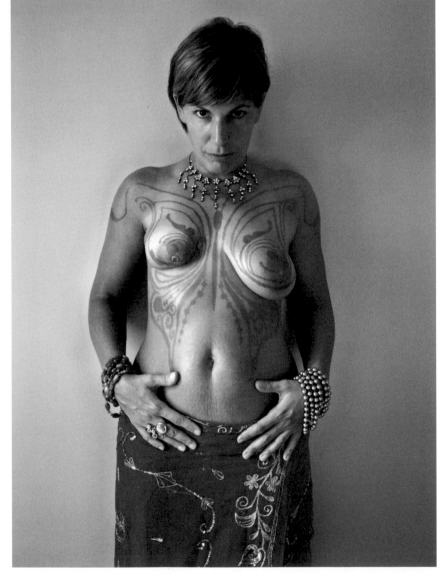

Pierrette

The photographer's sister, Pierrette Huberdeau, in September 2003. The previous year, Pierrette received the stunning diagnosis that she had cancer. "She got through her chemo and radiation quietly," says Denis. "She asked me to take her photo. She cried."

Photographer
Denis Levesque-Huberdeau
Montreal

Nathalie

Nathalie Ferron's doctors decided to operate two years after discovering a lump in her right breast, fearful that it may be cancerous. In this photo, Nathalie shows the anguish she went through while waiting for the results, which thankfully came back negative. "I understood what it was like to rub shoulders with cancer," she says.

Photographer
Nathalie Ferron
Gatineau

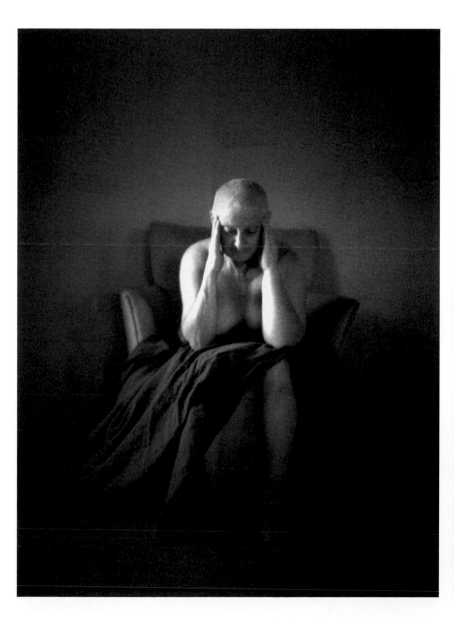

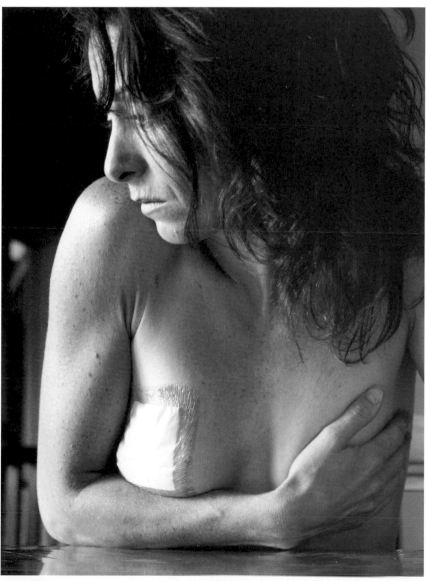

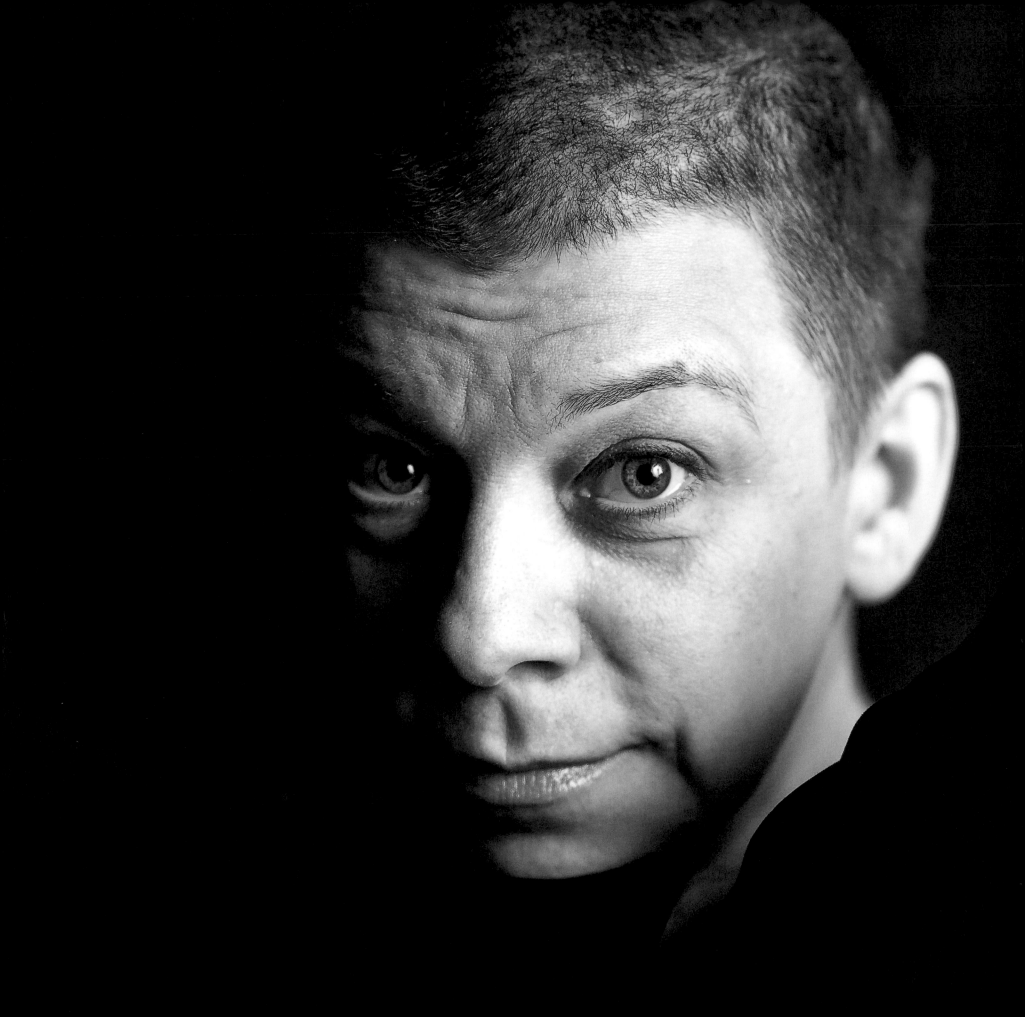

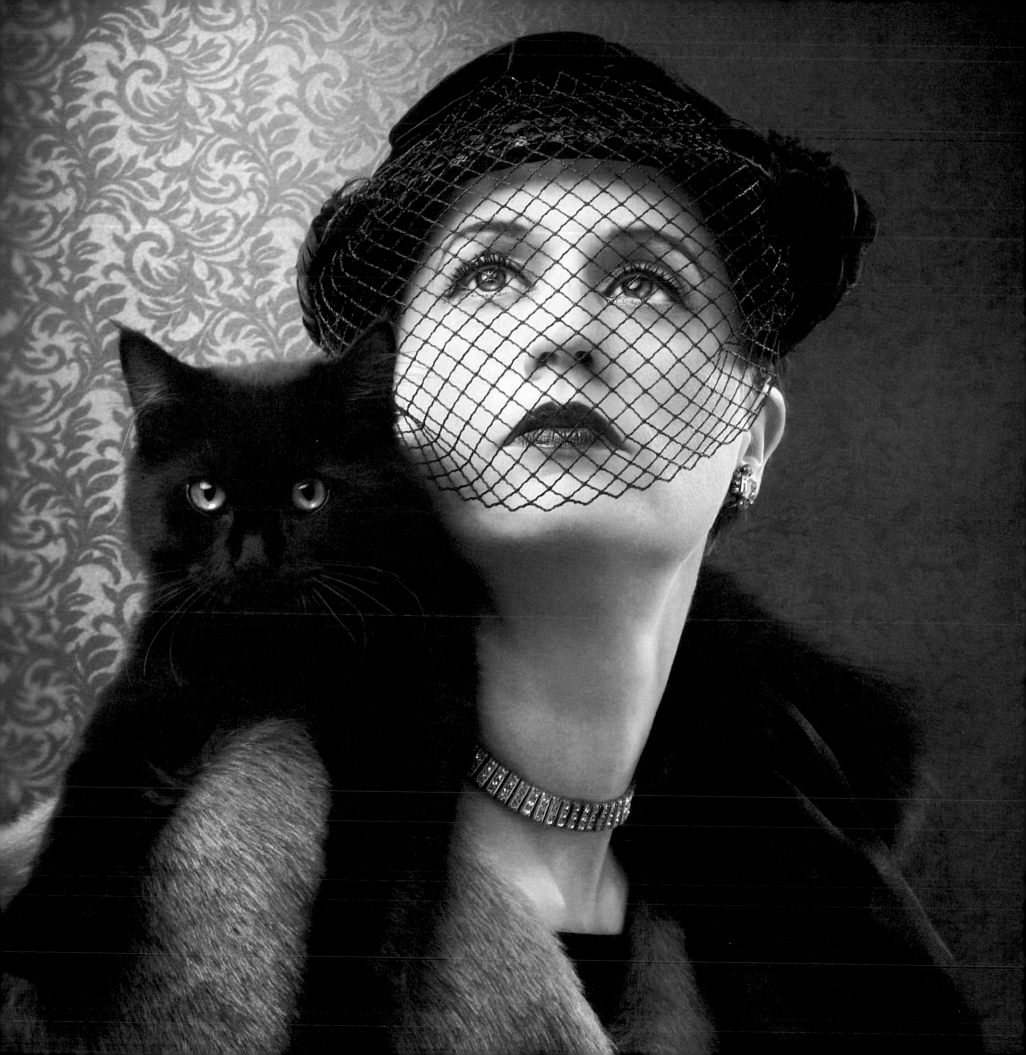

Previous left

Josée

Josée Bourdon was diagnosed with breast cancer in 2007. This picture was taken a few days after her first chemotherapy session, which followed two operations. She asked her husband to take a picture of her as proof to herself that she was still alive and pretty.

Photographer
Stéphane Gauthier
Montreal

Previous right

Elizabeth

Self-portrait of Elizabeth Knox, photographer, diagnosed with stage 2B breast cancer in 2007 at age 36. Subsequent to diagnosis, Elizabeth followed holistic healing modalities. She underwent a mastectomy and lymph node dissection but declined chemotherapy. Elizabeth considered herself cancer-free following surgery and wholeheartedly believes that attitude is paramount in healing.

Photographer
Elizabeth Knox
Montreal

Mireille

Actress Mireille Deyglun saw her father, brother, and two cousins die of lung cancer. After these events, her dog Max became a faithful companion and "therapist" to help her overcome her grief. Max has been and remains a source of joy and comfort for Mireille.

Photographer
Claire Beaugrand-
Champagne
Montreal

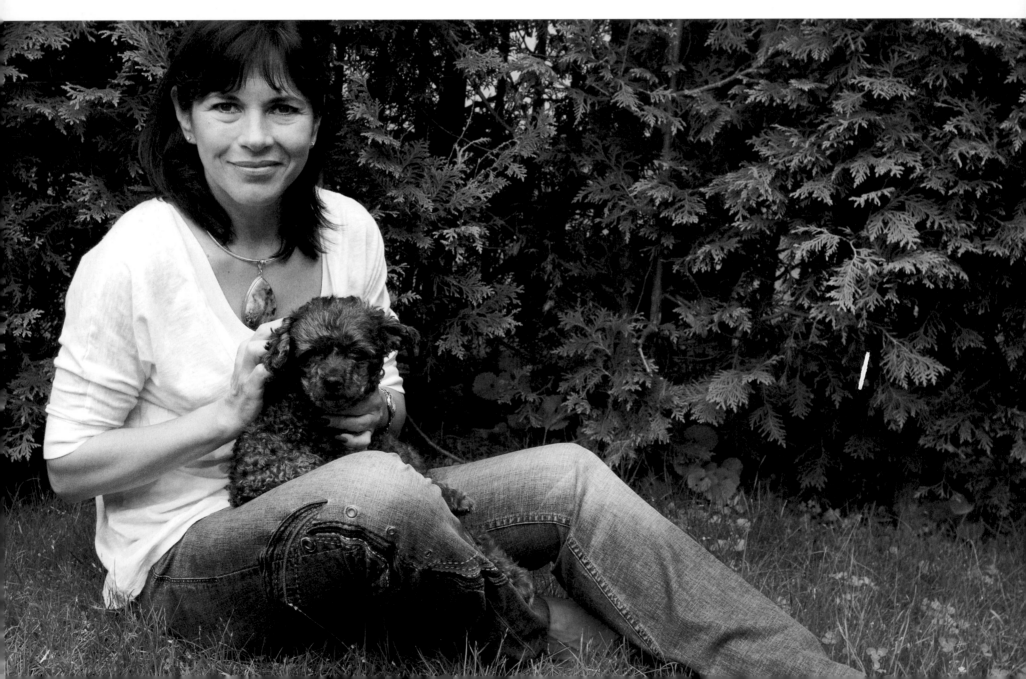

Rose Marie

In 2006, the photographer's mother, Rose Marie Stano, was diagnosed with a rare and aggressive form of melanoma. Today, she proudly wears her scar as a badge of courage.

Photographer
Kathy Slamen
St. Laurent

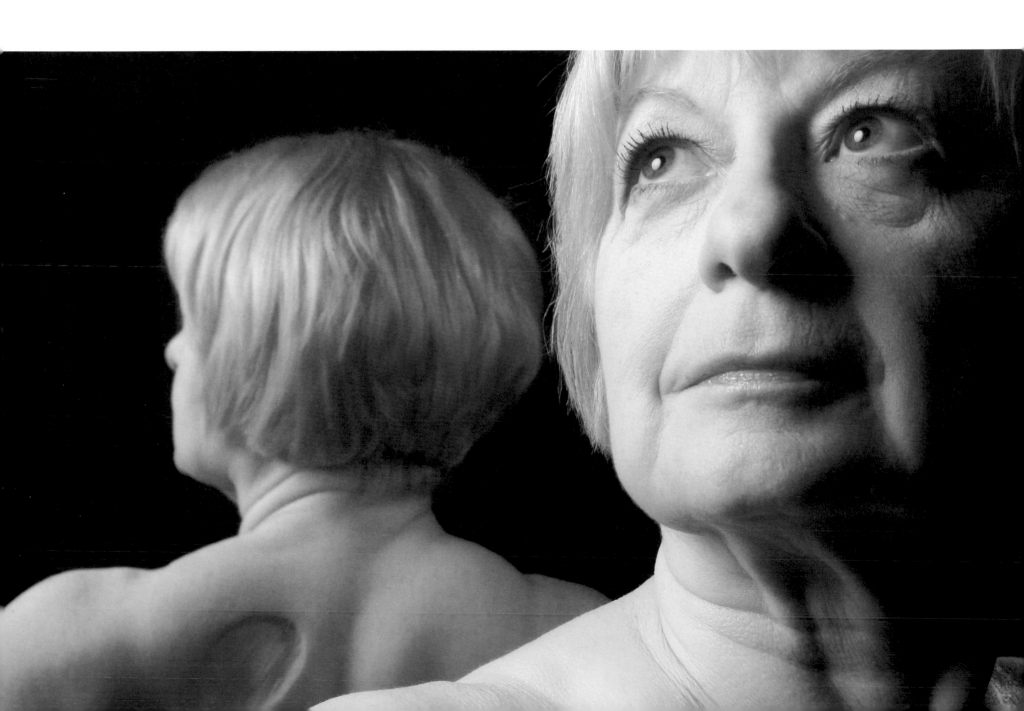

Renée

"Beauty of a mutilated body":
Renée Martin and friends
united against the disease.
Renée was diagnosed with
a very aggressive form
of breast cancer: her choice
was a mastectomy or death.
She had the breast removed,
and then reconstructed.
"One in the eye for the
disease," says Renée.

Photographer
Elise Racine
Granby

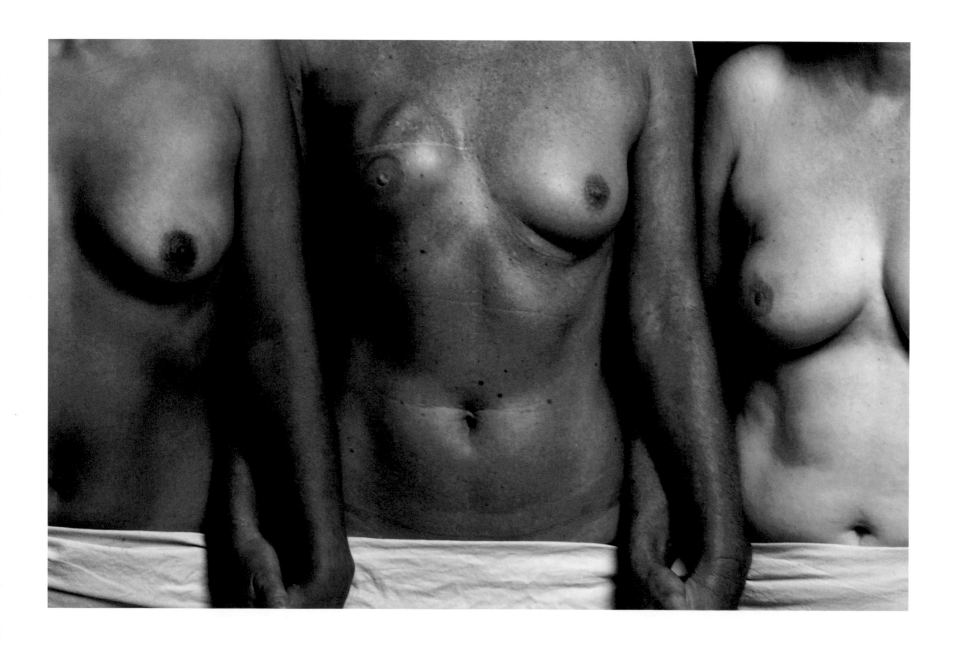

"May God give me the strength to live to see

the day when my daughter can live without suffering

from this disease."

Isabelle Massé

Betty and Emery

After putting on weight following radiation, Betty Esperanza, a three-time cancer survivor, wanted to free herself from a negative self-image. "Four years later and 50 pounds lighter, I celebrated by doing a nude photo session with my partner Emery. I am more than alive, I am immortal!"

Photographer
Karl Duarte
Westmount

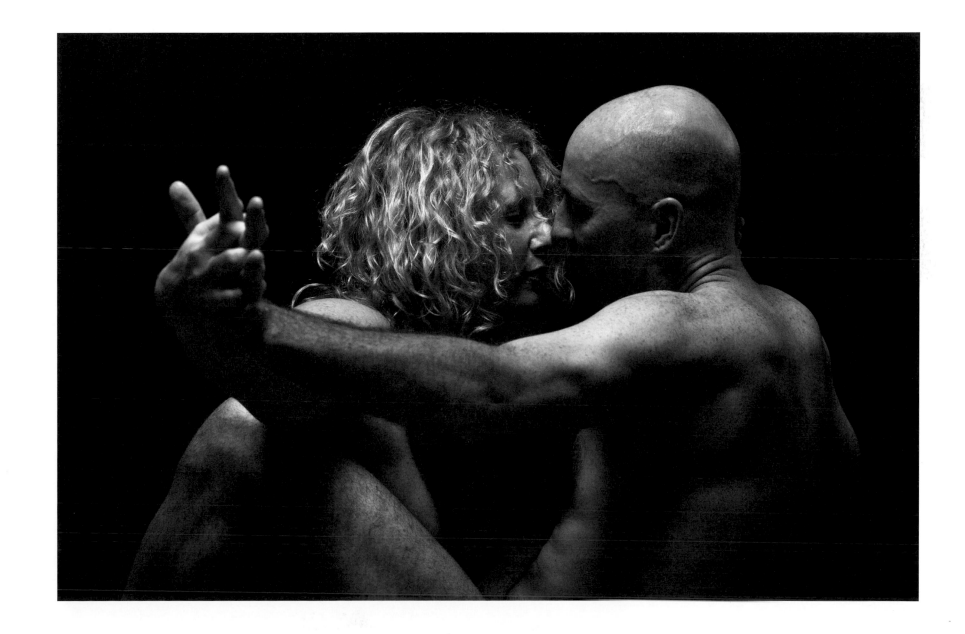

Gervais family

Five of eight siblings of the Gervais family, united in their fight against cancer. Lise, Dominique, Daniel, Michelle, and Claudette have all fought cancers, including breast, skin, Ewing's sarcoma, Hodgkin's disease, and basocellular carcinoma. Dominique is battling a second bout of breast cancer, while the rest are cancer-free or in remission.

Photographer
Jean-François Bérubé
Montreal

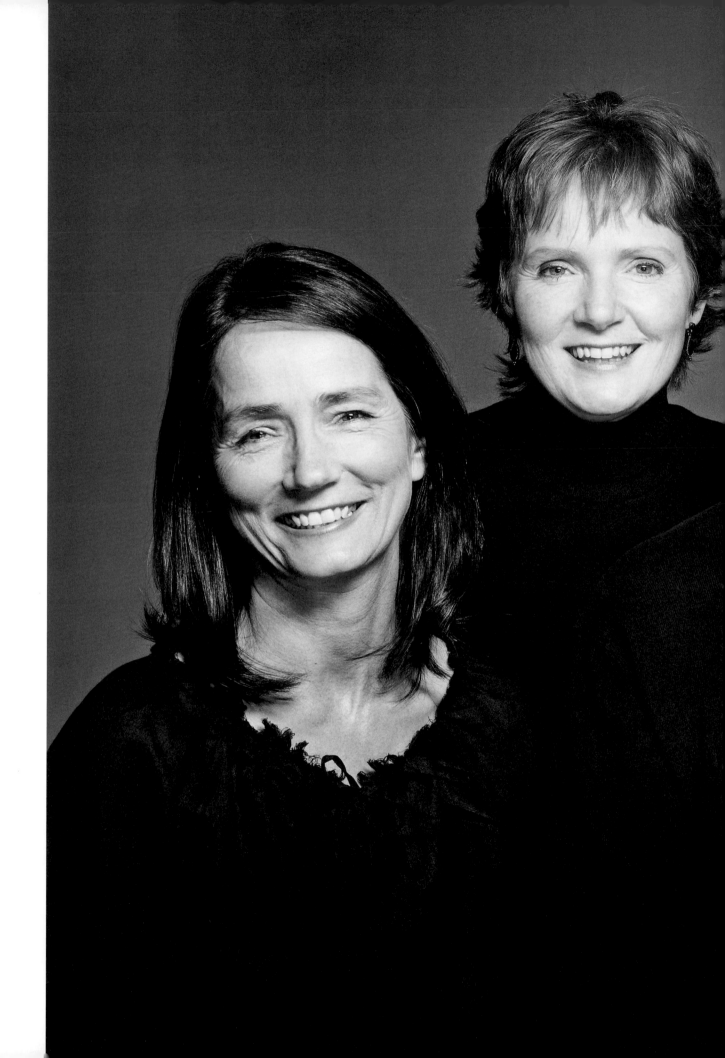

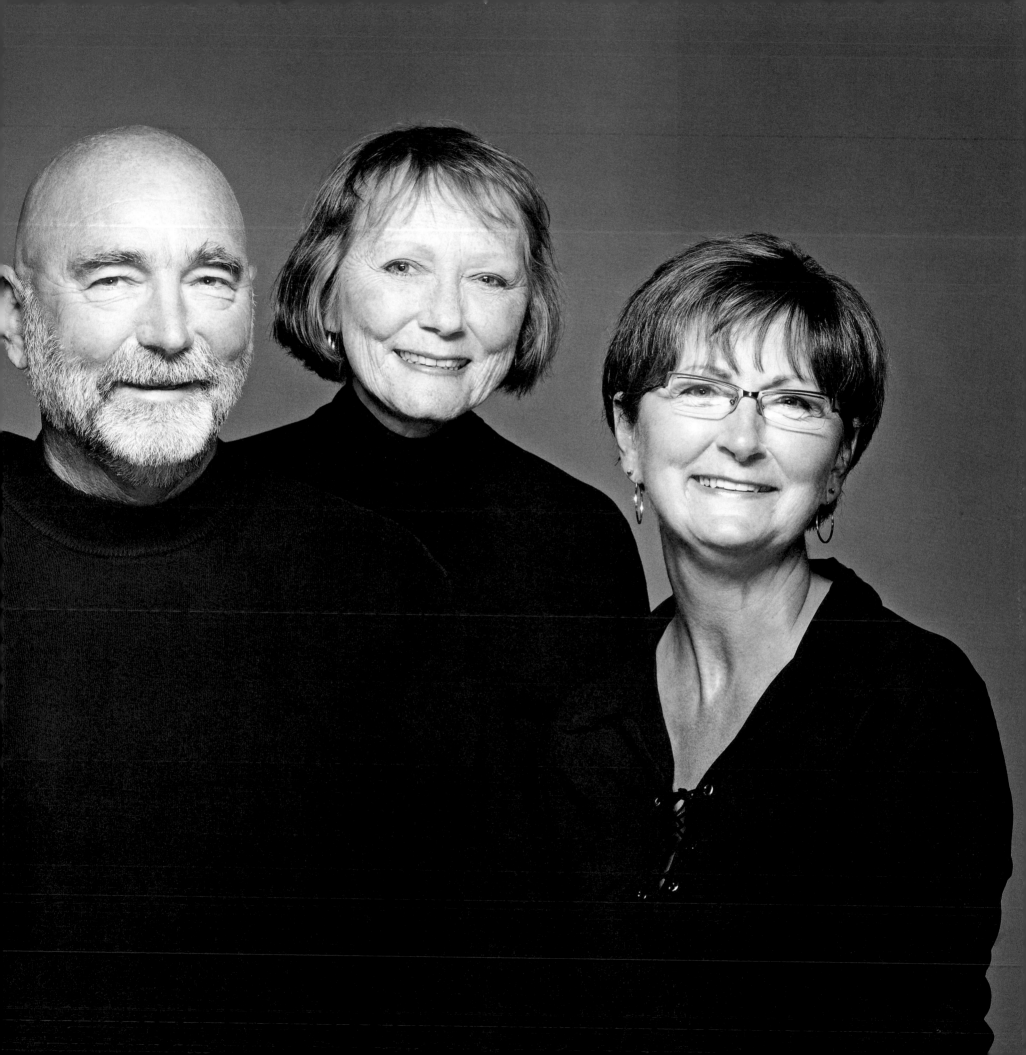

Row 1: Amélie Desrosiers, Laval; Andréanne Michon, Montreal; Bernard Brault, Longueuil; Bernard Charbonneau, Lasalle; Brigit-Alexandre Bussiere, Montreal; Camille Pasquin, Montreal; CaroH (7–8), Montreal

Row 2: CaroH, Montreal; Carole Guay, St-Jean-sur-Richelieu; Charles-Henri Debeur, Montreal; Christinne Muschi, Montreal; Christophe Hamelin, St. Bruno; Claudine Lahaie (6–7), Blue Sea; Claire Bolduc, Cantley

Row 3: Clement Beauregard, St-Basile-le-Grand; Danielle Gervais, Montreal; Diane Dupuis-Kallos, Montreal; Dominique Cantin, Montreal; Dorothy Dixon-Williams (5–7), Pierrefonds; Elise Racine, Granby

Row 4: Elizabeth Knox, Montreal; Francine Garneau (2–3), Gatineau; Gabriella Bruyere (4–6), St.Bruno; Gerald Beaudoin, Havelock; Guylaine Legault, St-Félix-De-Dalquier

Row 5: Jackie Cytrynbaum, Côte-St-Luc; Jena Martin, Montreal; Jean-François Dubé, Chicoutimi; Jennifer Piette, Chateauguay; Joan Sullivan (5–6), St. André Avelin; Johanne Sureau, Greenfield Park; Jonathan Clark, Montreal

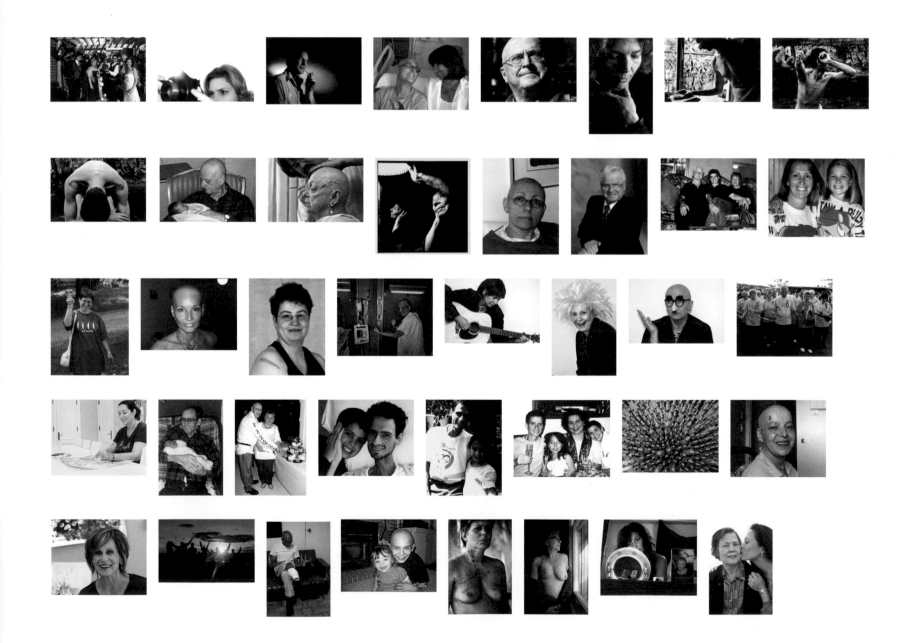

Row 1: Jonathan Taillefer, Longueuil; Katia Gosselin, Montreal; Kristi Kouchakji, Montreal; Line Lafantaisie, Laval; Lino Cipresso, St-Léonard; Lisa Graves, Montreal; Louis Avard, Ste-Adèle; Marc-André Pauzé, Winneway

Row 2: Marie-Claude Gaudet, Sainte-Geneviève-de-Batiscan; Marie-eve Bertrand, Montreal; Marilyn Jarrett, Montreal; Martin Chesnay, Montreal; Michael Leckman, Laval; Miguel Legault, Montreal; Nathalie Ferron, Gatineau

Row 3: Nathalie Ferron, Gatineau; Paul Fortier, St-Bruno-de-Montarville; Phil Carpenter, Greenfield Park; Réjean Duval, Montreal; Sara McCulloch, Montreal; Simon Lafreniere, Dorval; Vicky Vriniotis, Pierrefonds; Yann-Manuel Hernandez, Brossard

Row 4: Yves Choquette (1–2), Montreal

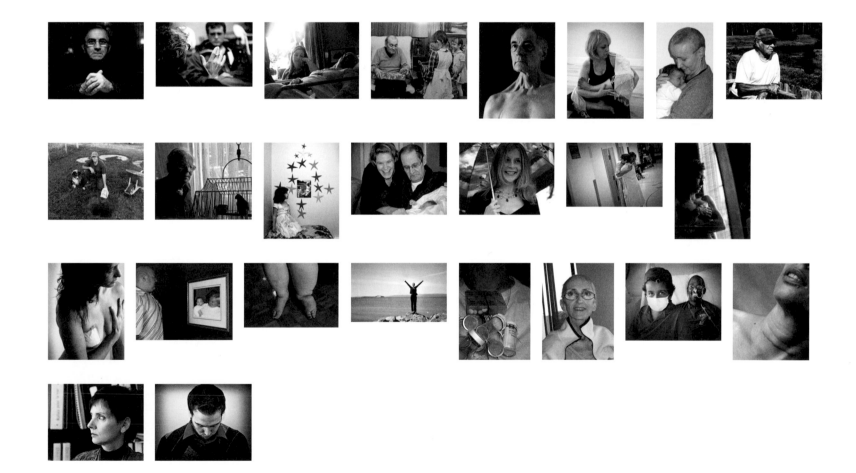

The Maritimes

New Brunswick, Newfoundland and Labrador,
Nova Scotia, and Prince Edward Island

"I realized I only get one life to live and once I'm through with it, that's it. I'll have had my chance."

Robin Maher

Photographer
Angela Butler
Mt. Pearl, Newfoundland
and Labrador

Angela

After being diagnosed with stage 3b Hodgkin's lymphoma on May 11, 2009, at age 17, Angela Butler took a photo every day of her cancer journey. This photo is entitled "There ain't no party like a Gallium scan part*ay*!"

"I love documenting things. I've done it my whole life," says Angela. "The first day I was diagnosed with cancer, I had my camera with me, as always, and I took a picture of my hospital wristband. I started posting on Flickr and it became like therapy for me. I would write about what was happening to me and post a photo along with it. It helped me to get my thoughts together."

Many of the self-portraits were taken at the Janeway Children's Hospital in St. John's, where Angela had her treatment. Online photos included images of her going through chemotherapy, tests, scans, and X-rays, and ways in which she got through the experience.

For Angela, the hardest part of the experience was dealing with the side effects of the chemotherapy. "After taking the chemo I would get pins and needles in my hands, arms, feet, and legs. I got it on and off for about three days straight. It was so painful I couldn't walk. I was in a wheelchair and needed help just to go to the bathroom. They put me on codeine but that didn't really help, and it got worse after every cycle."

Doctors changed her treatment to a different and more aggressive chemotherapy that didn't give her pins and needles, but did make her feel very sick. "That chemo really knocked me out. All I could do was sleep and then when I woke up, I would throw up."

In October 2009, Angela was told that the tumour had shrunk to almost nothing and that she was considered in remission. She immediately began a new photo-a-day project on Flickr— Project 365—which lasted a year.

"I didn't expect to finish my 365 here," says Angela, speaking of her new home at the Alberta College of Art and Design. "A lot of good things came out of my cancer experience. I met a lot of great people through Flickr, including Kay Burns, who encouraged me to apply to the best arts schools in Canada. She helped me get into ACAD, where I've just started a four-year course."

The cancer remains in the back of Angela's mind and she still has physical side effects from the chemotherapy. "I always think about the cancer, but not to the point where it distracts me from doing other things."

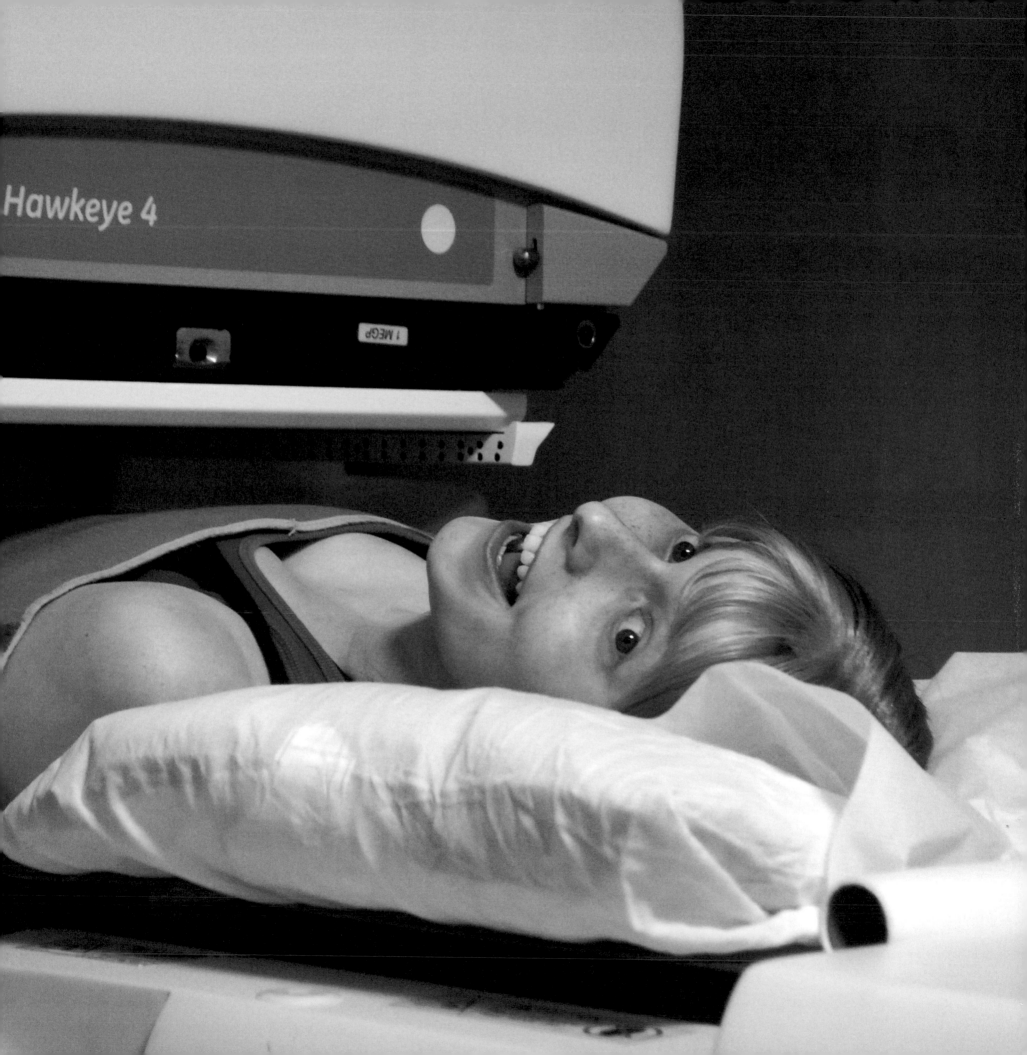

Shauna

Shauna MacLean on a beach
soon after learning that
the breast cancer that she
had been battling was gone.
She says, "This was a way
to celebrate life. I like
to refer to it as the calm
after the storm."

Photographer
John Ratchford
River Ryan, Nova Scotia

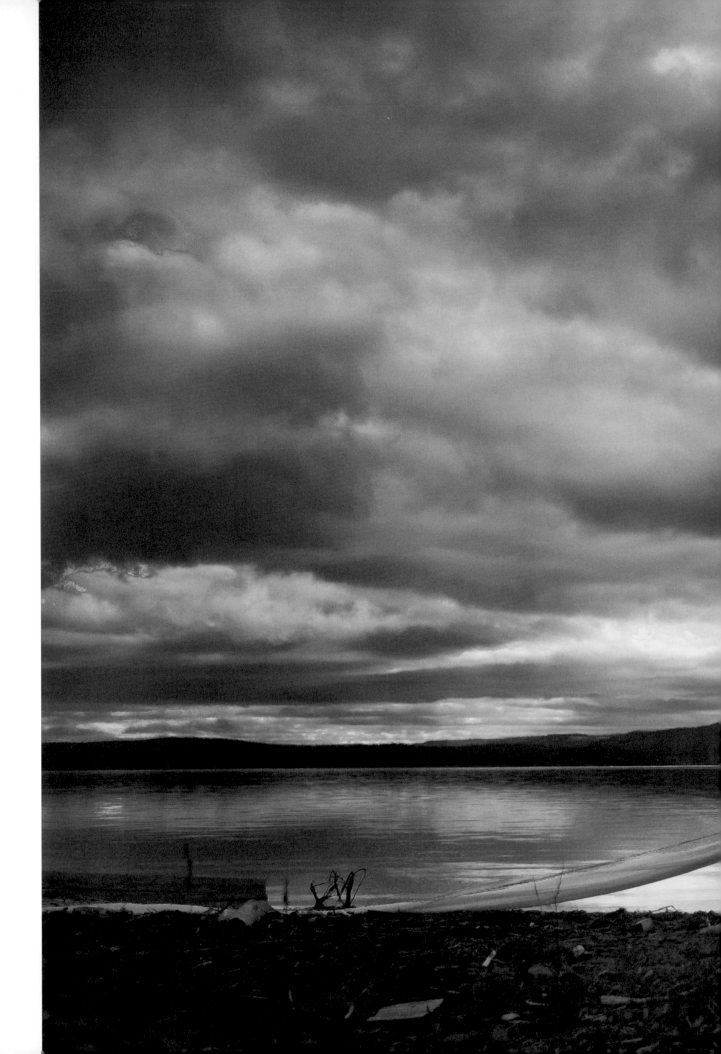

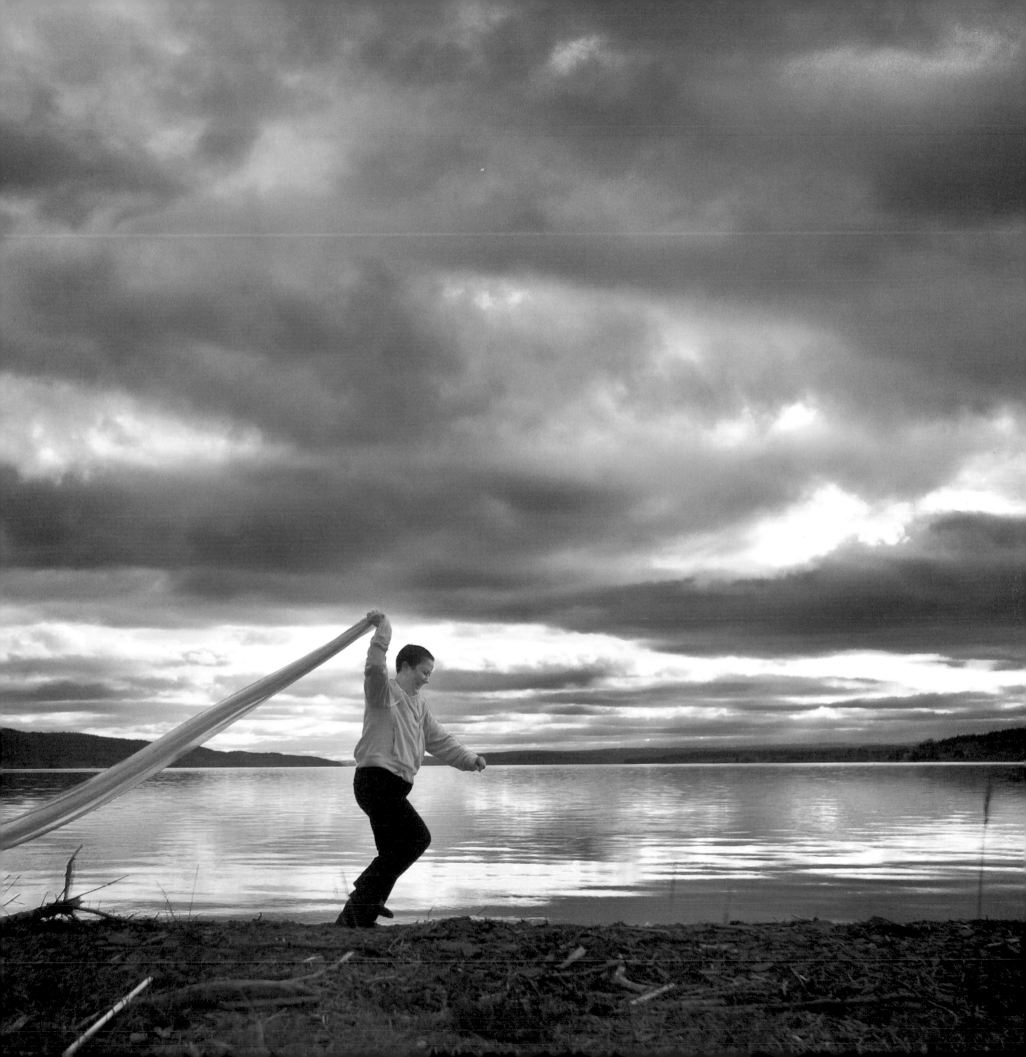

Anne

Anne Duguay, diagnosed with ductal carcinoma in situ, photographed the day before her mastectomy surgery. Anne lost a sister to breast cancer some years ago. At the shoot she said, "I want a picture of myself with my real twins one last time."

Photographer
Georges Long
Fredericton,
New Brunswick

Nora

Nova Scotia artist Nora Gross, a breast cancer survivor, after recently undergoing a mastectomy. To show her artistic connection, she is painted with a butterfly design, and to show her bravery and joy of life, she is photographed showing her scars.

Photographer
Shari Tucker
Dartmouth, Nova Scotia

Opposite

Melanie

Melanie Roach was only 25 when she discovered she had breast cancer. After a mastectomy, chemotherapy, and hormonal therapy, she is now cancer-free. Melanie says, "The hardest part at the time was losing my hair because it was such a part of my identity and femininity. Cancer has taught me that no matter what life throws at me, I will be able to deal with it."

Photographer
John Ratchford
Glace Bay, Nova Scotia

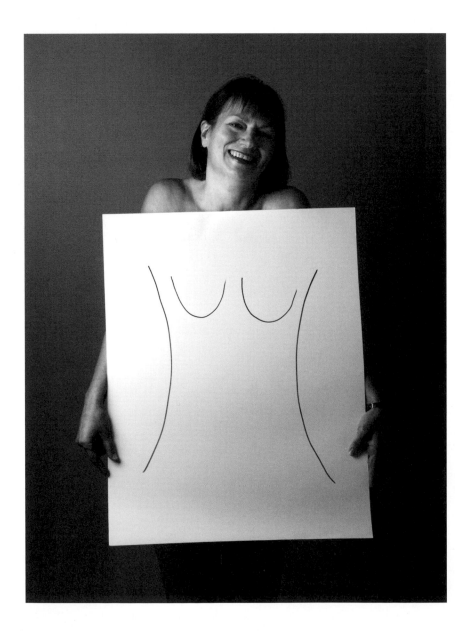

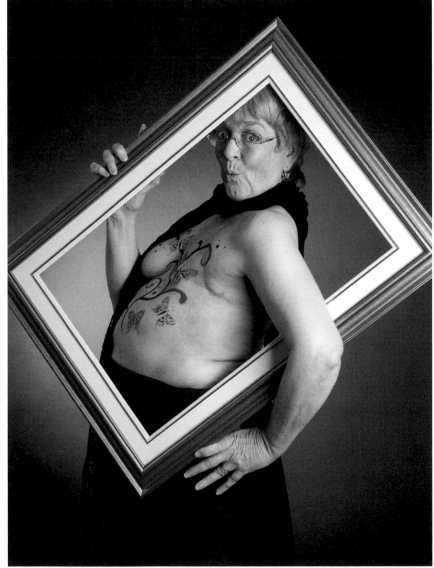

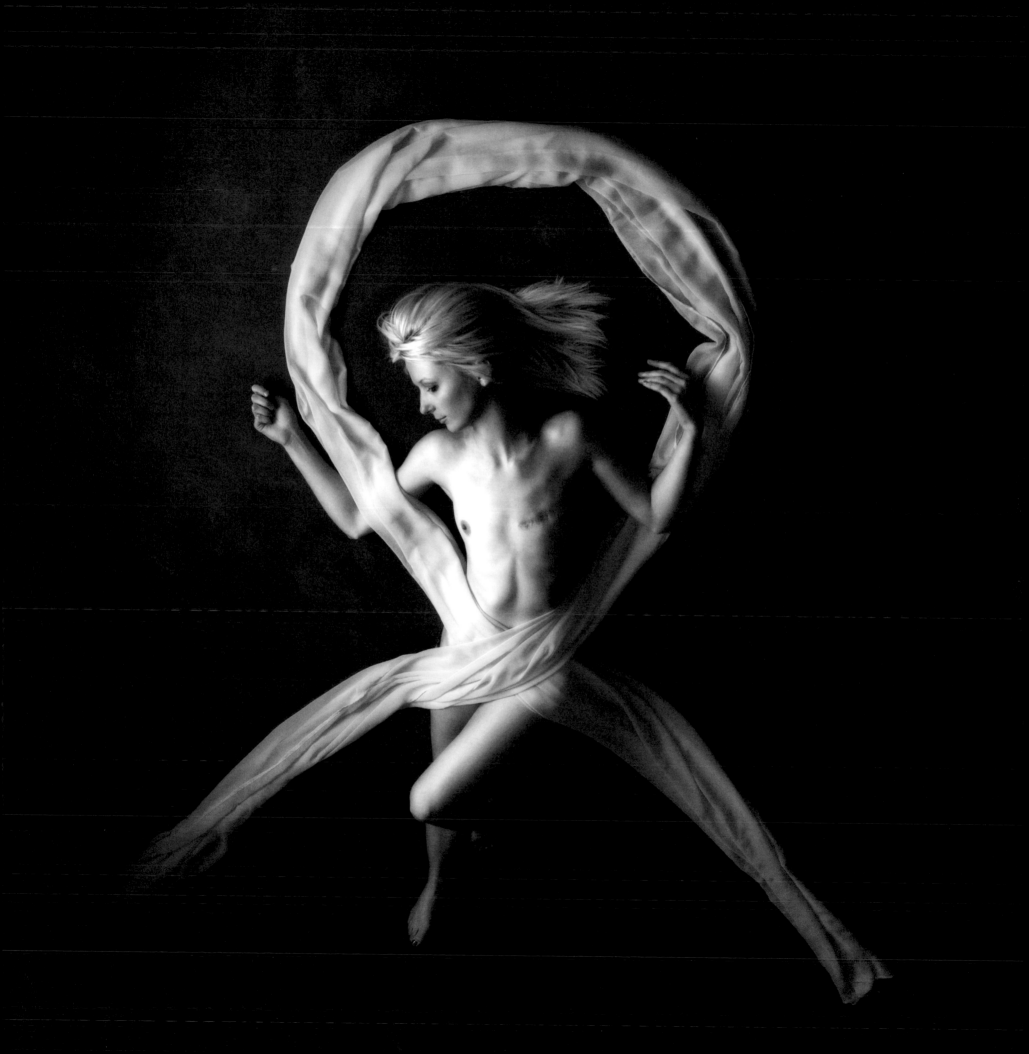

Gary

Gary was given a bleak prognosis in 1998 when first diagnosed with a rare form of cancer. He has had several operations to remove large and small tumours and has had his right leg amputated. He is still fighting the disease. Gary continues to golf, preferring to play without the hindrance of his prosthetic leg.

Photographer
Diane Slaunwhite
Dartmouth, Nova Scotia

Malcolm

When he was 10, Malcolm found a lump in his throat and went for a biopsy. The diagnosis was non-Hodgkin's Burkitt's lymphoma, which had spread to his liver, shin bones, and spine. After intense treatment, which made him feel extremely sick, Malcolm recovered fully. He is now back playing soccer, hockey, and other sports.

Photographer
Matthew Thompson
Sackville, New Brunswick

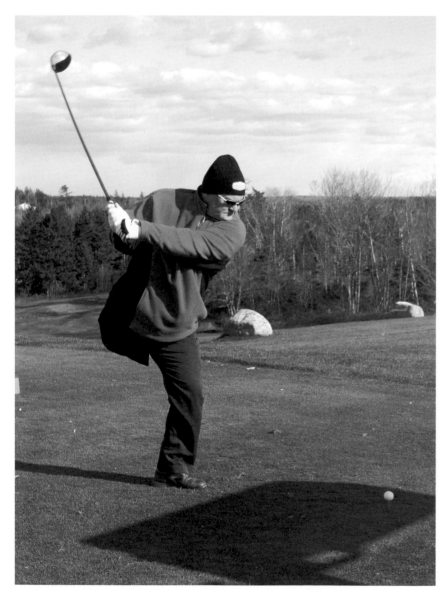

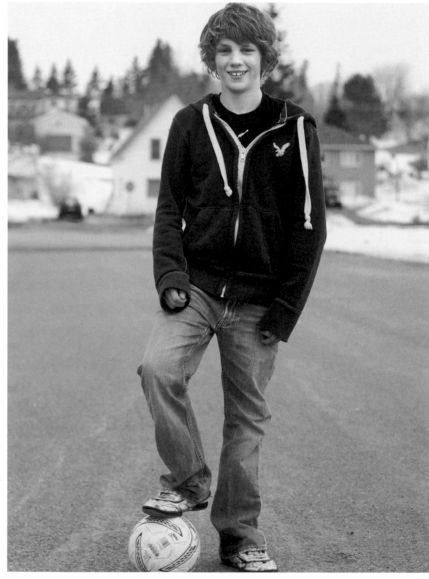

Ryan

Now 27, Ryan Joudrey has been cancer-free for over five years. Although shy at times, he was determined to overcome the obstacles facing him during his fight with acute lymphocytic leukemia. He says, "I sincerely doubt I would be alive today without the love and support of family, friends, doctors, and nurses."

Photographer
Shari Tucker
Halifax, Nova Scotia

Brad

At the age of six, Brad was diagnosed with rhabdomyo-sarcoma (a fast-growing, highly malignant tumour that accounts for over half of the soft tissue sarcomas in children). After over 60 treatments of radiation, 25 chemotherapy sessions, and 10 surgeries, he is now cancer-free.

Photographer
Nate Gates
Goulds, Newfoundland and Labrador

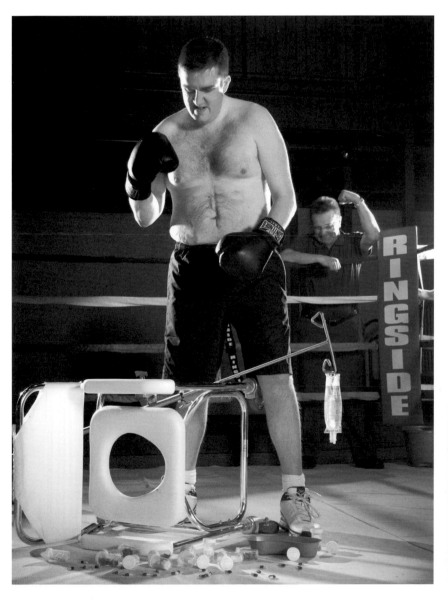

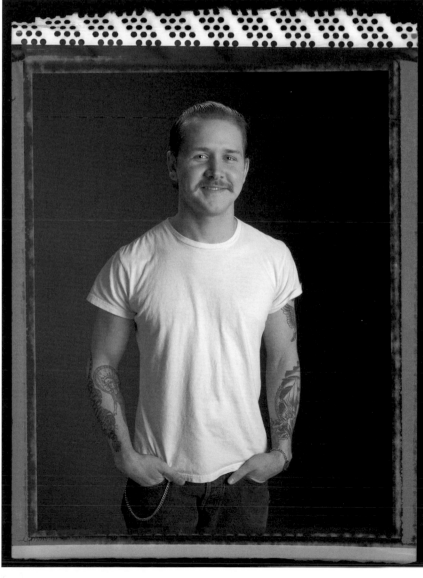

Photographer
Martin Flewwelling
Saint John, New Brunswick

Jim

Jim Brittain, a prostate cancer survivor, was one of several men who took off their pants to raise awareness about the disease and advertise the Saint John (New Brunswick) Regional Hospital Foundation's Rally of Hope. The 2008 rally supported a project to treat prostate cancer. The poster read: *I'm taking off my pants to get you talking.*

"Even today," says Jim, "people come up to me and say, 'Oh, it's nice to see you with your pants on.'" But in spite of the campaign's levity, it carried a serious message.

"Men don't talk to each other about their health," says Jim. "They do not go for regular PSAs, and they do not do what they are supposed to do, because they are macho and tough and think that nothing bad is going to happen to them. One of the reasons why this picture was published and got so much promotion was that we wanted to shock men into thinking, 'I need to look after myself, I should be doing what I need to be doing.'"

Thankfully, Jim had been doing what he should be doing for many years. When his regular PSA (prostate-specific antigen) tests showed that the number had risen from four to nine, his urologist told him they needed to do something about it. After reading a book on prostate cancer and being advised that his disease had

an 80 per cent chance of being completely confined to his prostate, Jim's response was immediate: "It's a no-brainer. Get it out, get it out as quickly as you can."

After the operation, Jim was given a clean bill of health, with no sign of the cancer having spread, no lymph nodes affected, and no further treatment required.

Unfortunately, less than two years later, Jim's PSAs started going up again and he was referred to an oncologist, who initiated an immediate regime of hormone therapy and radiation treatment.

"The doctors believed that the tumour was being fed by testosterone, so the idea was that the hormone treatment would tell my testes to stop producing it. Every time I had a hot flash, I'd say, 'Here we go again,' and my wife would look at me and smile and say, 'I told you what it's like and now you know!'"

Apart from some minor side effects, Jim recovered well after the second round of treatment. "I'm feeling as good as I did before I got sick. I have regular PSA checks and they've been fine. There's nothing you could put your finger on that would make you think that I've experienced cancer."

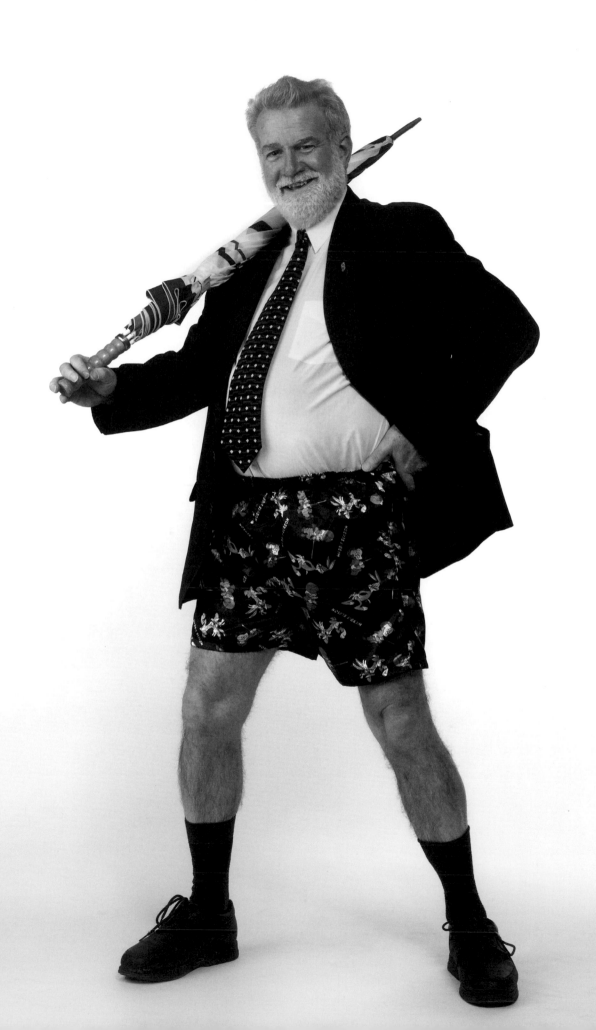

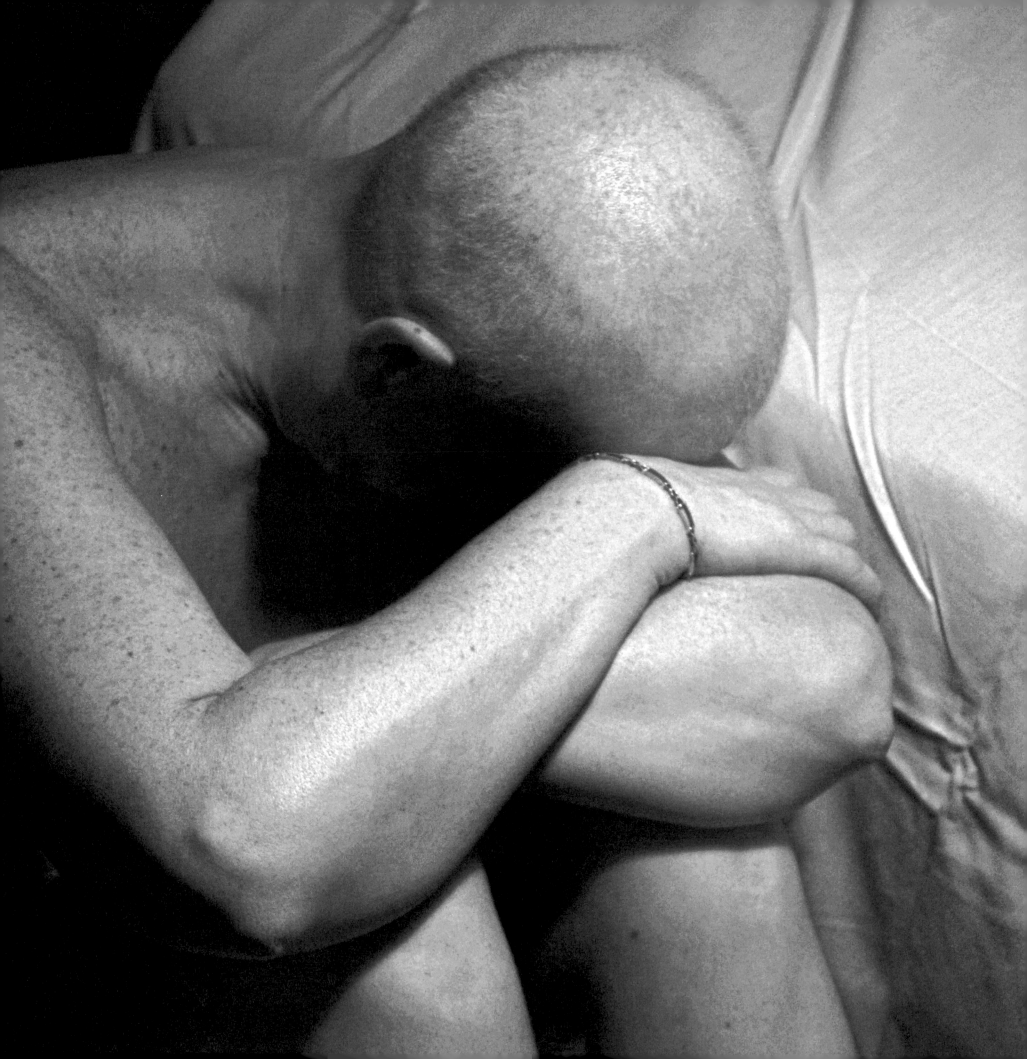

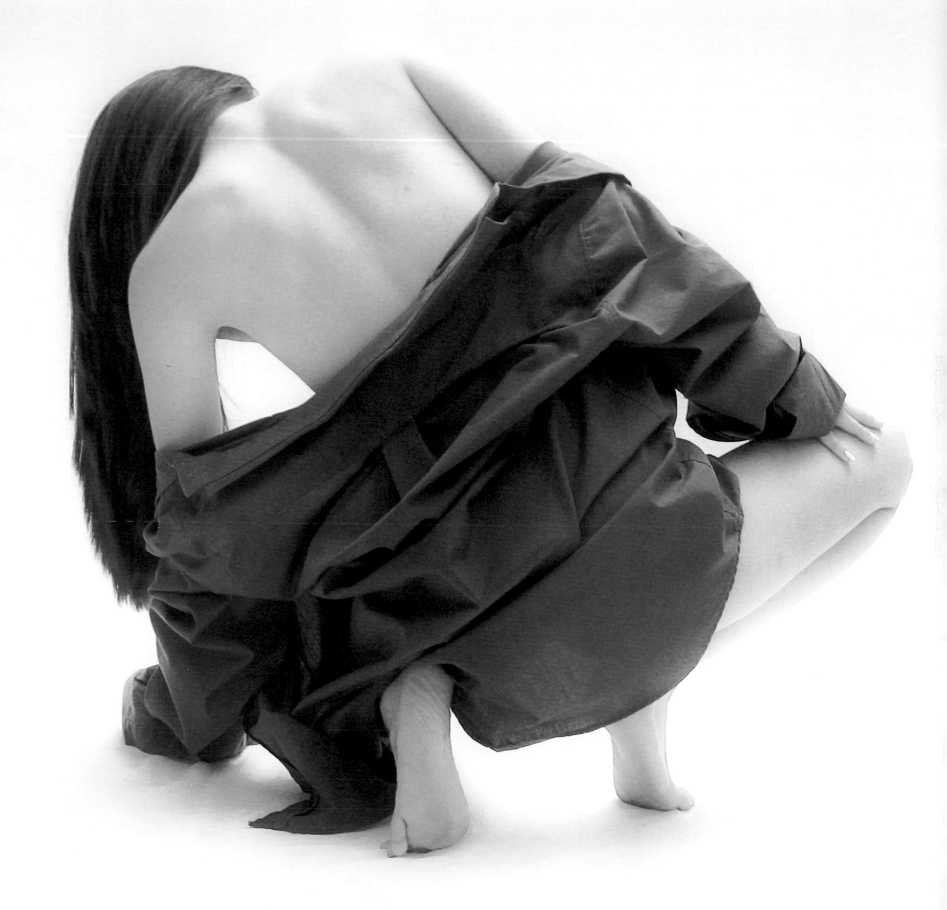

Previous left

Trudy

Après chemo: Trudy, photographer Lisa's good friend. "When she was diagnosed with breast cancer, it was a shock to everyone," says Lisa. Lisa was hesitant to ask if she could take Trudy's photograph post-chemo, but then Trudy asked if Lisa would. "She's feeling great now, for which we are all truly grateful."

Photographer
Lisa Piercey
St. John's, Newfoundland
and Labrador

Previous right

Andrea

Andrea discovered she had cancer after preliminary examinations for breast enhancement. Sometimes she's frightened by the spiders she hallucinates about due to her pain-killers. Although treatment has meant quitting her business and university, she is happy and optimistic, and has recently found love.

Photographer
Hugo J. Bohorquez
Halifax, Nova Scotia

Dan and Linda

When Dan was diagnosed with cancer, he had to travel several times to St. John's, Newfoundland, for treatment. Coming from a small, coastal community in Labrador, he and his wife, Linda, found the culture shock challenging, with the difference in lifestyle making them feel isolated and alone.

Photographer
Sheilagh O'Leary
Rigolet, Newfoundland
and Labrador

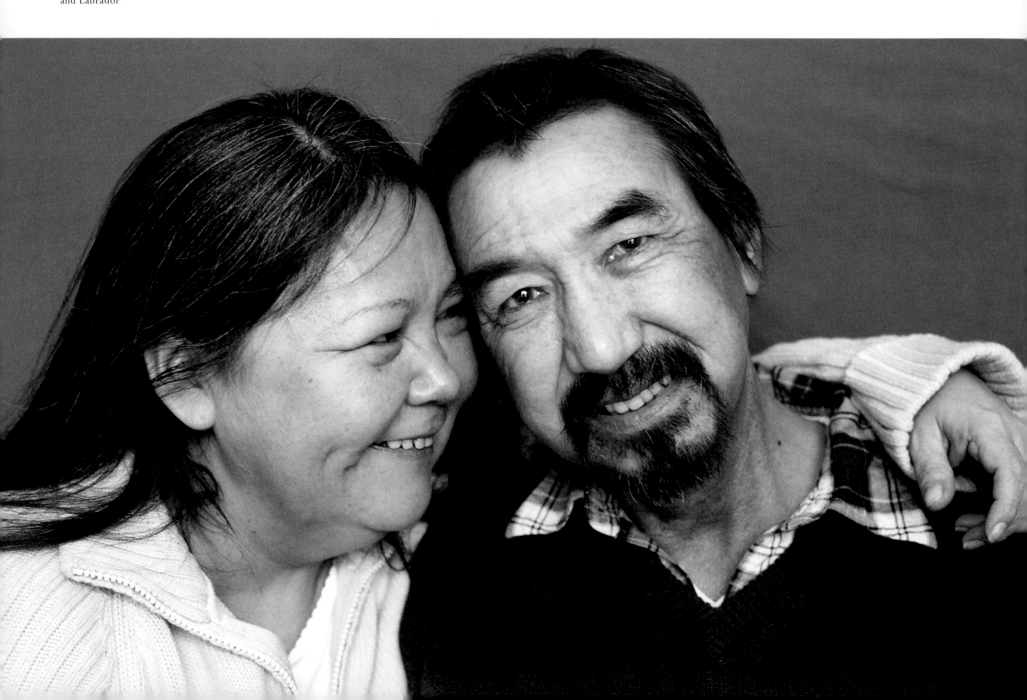

Chuck and Ryan

Chuck, with his son Ryan.
After being diagnosed with
squamous cell carcinoma
in 2003, Chuck had to spend
so much time in St. John's
that he ended up buying an
apartment in the city. Chuck
has now been in remission
for over five years.

Photographer
Sheilagh O'Leary
Goose Bay, Newfoundland
and Labrador

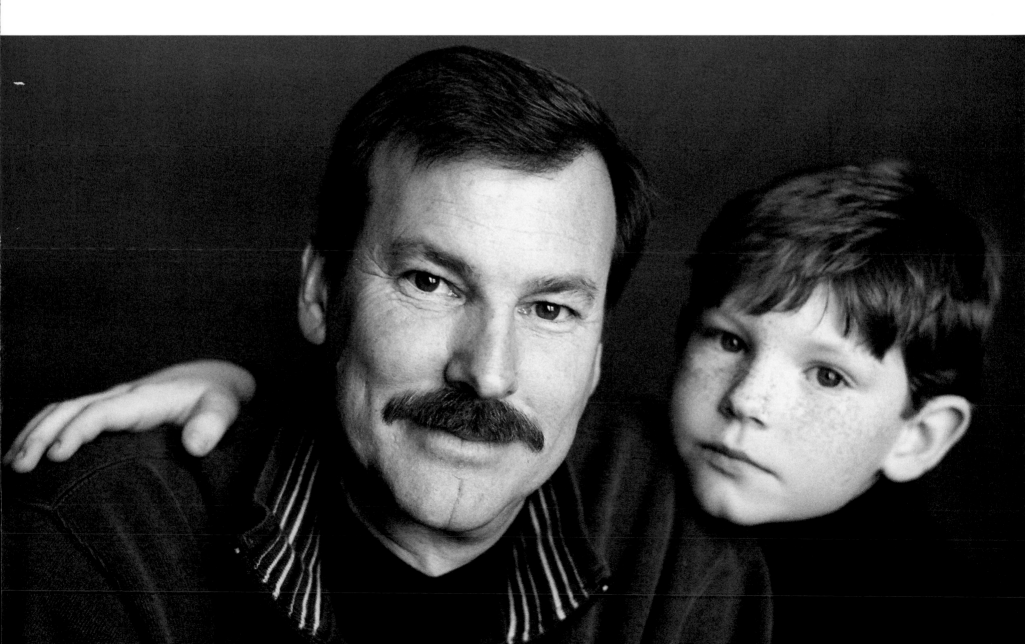

Robin

When she was 15, Robin Maher was sick for months and misdiagnosed before finally discovering that she had Hodgkin's lymphoma. Now 22 and well, she says, "I honestly appreciate every day. I realize I only get one life to live and once I'm through with it, that's it, I'll have had my chance."

Photographer
Shari Tucker
Antigonish, Nova Scotia

Gabriel

Gabriel was diagnosed with acute myeloid leukemia when he was just over 10 months old. Six months of treatment, an incredibly supportive family, and lots of encouragement helped him to kick the disease. His family is thankful to have Gabriel with them and enjoys small blessings like being able to play with him in the park.

Photographer
Shari Tucker
New Glasgow, Nova Scotia

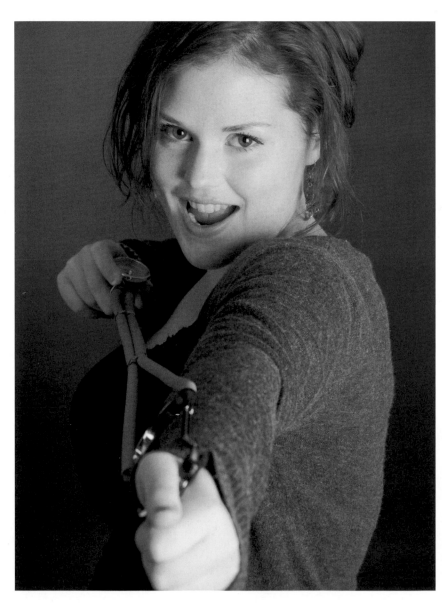

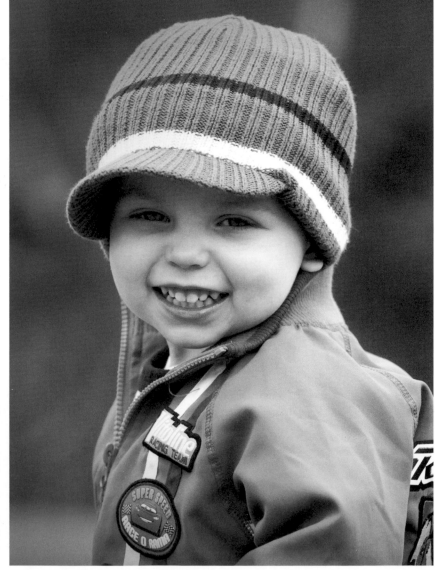

Jillian

Jillian, soon after being diagnosed with stage 3 neuroblastoma at 21 months of age. After chemotherapy and surgery she recovered and is now a vibrant and healthy nine-year-old. "All you need is hope," says Jillian's mother, photographer Bernadette.

Photographer
Bernadette Morris
Hammonds Plains,
Nova Scotia

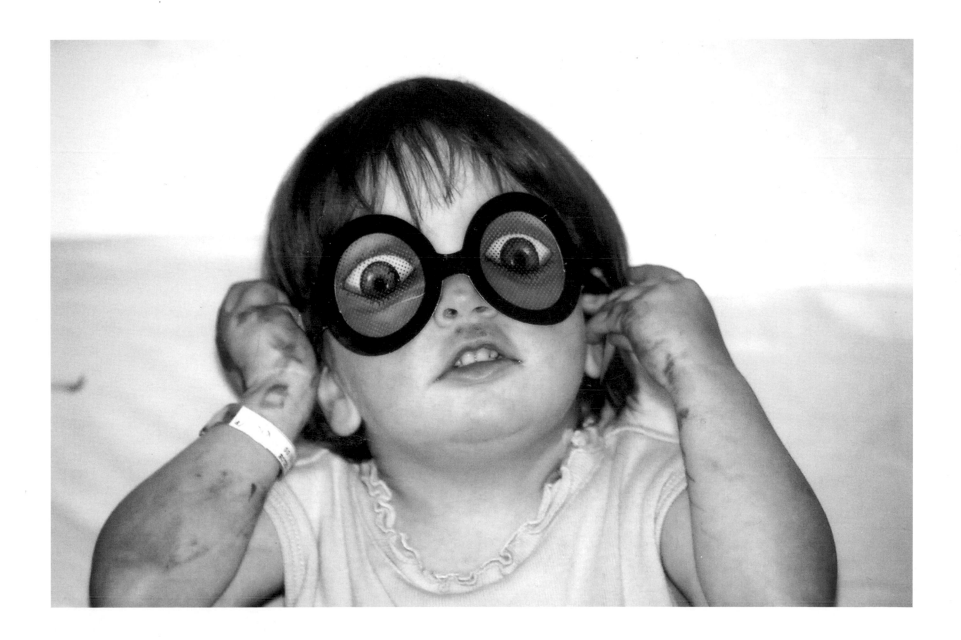

Ok bud, now that I've gotten over the initial shock:
The shot has an eerie beauty to it.
It's you, facing it all head-on,
as you have gone with foes in the past.
As much as I associated the curly mop-top
with you, Liz, after a few seconds I was ok with
the mop-top not being there.
It's all good, Bud.
That is still your beautiful face,
those are still your beautiful eyes,
your soul
shining through.
Your fight
shining through
want to say
it's a brave shot.

but
it's way beyond that.

Thank you for trusting me,
for letting me in that far.
You know
I'll always
be here for you.

Love
Frank

Opposite

Liz

Liz Curran's gynecologist was amazed when he diagnosed her with endometrial cancer in 2009, because she wasn't post-menopausal, a smoker, or obese. Liz says, "I know I am lucky to have dedicated and caring medical professionals and friends and family that demonstrate their endless love to me every day."

Photographer
Liz Curran
Fall River, Nova Scotia

Judy

Photographer Liam Hennessey struggled to talk about his feelings when his mother, Judy, was battling cancer, so he agreed to photograph her last chemotherapy session. Liam says, "The result is a collection of raw, real, and imperfect images that show the reality of it all. It was an overwhelming experience for our whole family. These days we celebrate Mom's remission."

Photographer
Liam Hennessey
Boutiliers Point, Nova Scotia

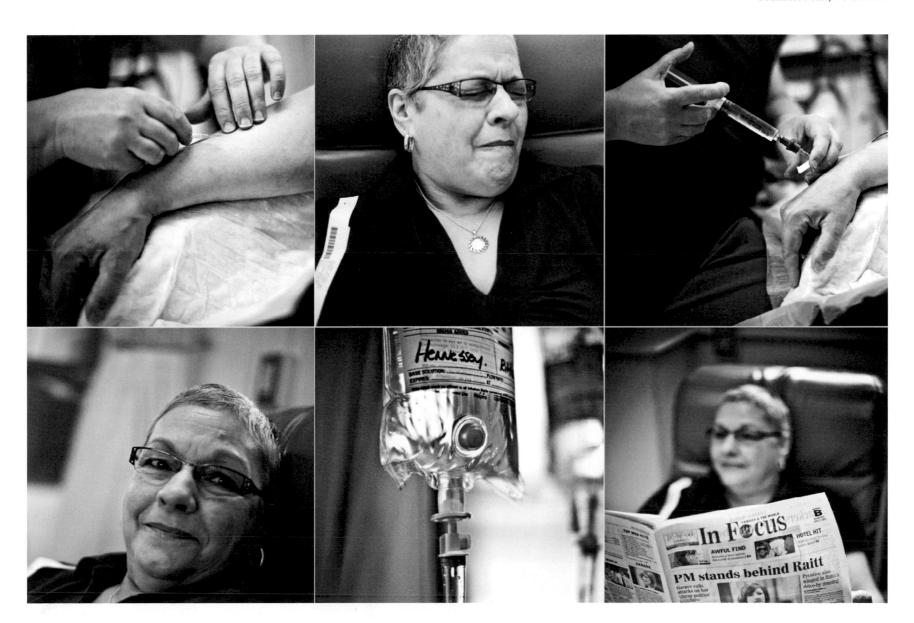

Row 1: Alanna Jankov, Charlottetown, Prince Edward Island; Alex MacAulay, Halifax, Nova Scotia; Andre Reinders, Saint John, New Brunswick; Angela Butler (4–8), Mt. Pearl, Newfoundland and Labrador

Row 2: Bernadette Morris (1–3), Hammonds Plains, Nova Scotia; Denise Rowe (4–8), Fredericton, New Brunswick

Row 3: Diane Slaunwhite, Dartmouth, Nova Scotia; Ed Boulter, Beaver Bank, Nova Scotia; Elizabeth Spencer, Cooks Brook, Nova Scotia; Erin Kelly, Saint John, New Brunswick; Gavin Simms, Port Union, Newfoundland and Labrador; Georges Long (6–8), Fredericton, New Brunswick

Row 4: Heather Dominie, Ramea, Newfoundland and Labrador; Heather Kirby, Halifax, Nova Scotia; Heather Sproat (3–4), Moncton, New Brunswick; Hilda Cousins, St. John's, Newfoundland and Labrador; James Burns, Halifax, Nova Scotia; James Helmer, Truro, Nova Scotia; Jim Day, Charlottetown, Prince Edward Island

Row 5: Joel Jacobson, Halifax, Nova Scotia; John Ratchford (2–5), River Ryan, Nova Scotia; John Sylvester, (6–7), Charlottetown, Prince Edward Island; Joseph Chater, Halifax, Nova Scotia

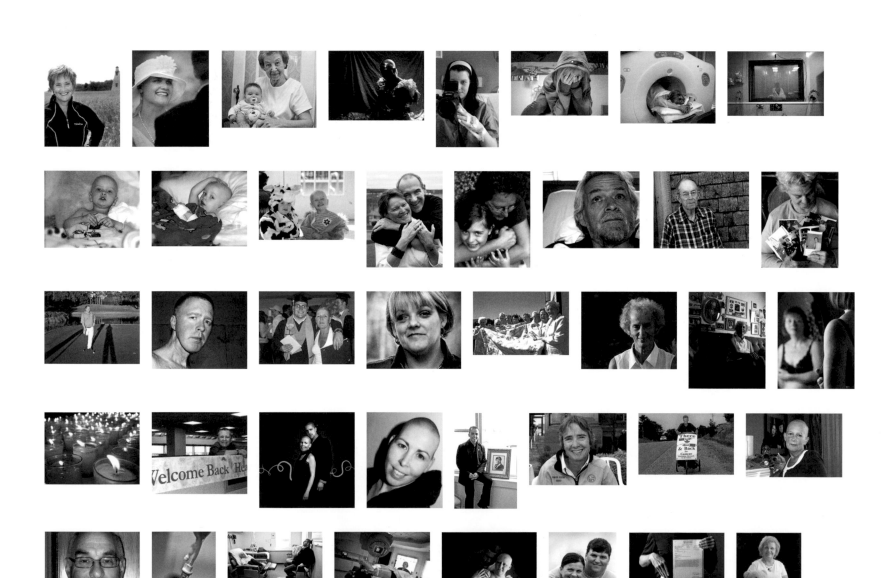

Row 1: Joseph Chater, Halifax, Nova Scotia; Karine Thériault, Dartmouth, Nova Scotia; Karla Kenny, St. John's, Newfoundland and Labrador; Kevin Hoyt, Arviat, Nunavut; Kylie Churchill, St. John's, Newfoundland and Labrador; Linda Morehouse, Fredericton, New Brunswick; Lolek Morawiecki, Cape Breton, Nova Scotia; Lynn Butler, Bedford, Nova Scotia

Row 2: Marc Xavier LeBlanc (1–2), Moncton, New Brunswick; Martin Flewwelling, Saint John, New Brunswick; Marty Melanson, Moncton, New Brunswick; Matthew Thompson (5–6), Sackville, New Brunswick; Mike Little, Halifax, Nova Scotia; Nigel Armstrong, Charlottetown, Prince Edward Island

Row 3: Norm Lewicki, Mazerolle Settlement, New Brunswick; Pat Le Clair, Charlottetown, Prince Edward Island; Paul Daly (3–4), St. John's, Newfoundland and Labrador; Phil Carpenter, Quispamsis, New Brunswick; Pierre Fortier, Halifax, Nova Scotia; Sandor Fizli (7–8), South Brook, Newfoundland and Labrador

Row 4: Sandor Fizli (1–2), South Brook, Newfoundland and Labrador; Shanie Stozek, Beresford, New Brunswick; Shari Tucker (4–8), Lower Sackville, Nova Scotia

Row 5: Sheilagh O'Leary (1–2), Labrador City, Newfoundland and Labrador; Sheilagh O'Leary, Corner Brook, Newfoundland and Labrador; Stephanie O'Neill (4–5), Herring Cove, Nova Scotia; Teri Johnson, Dartmouth, Nova Scotia; Tracy Boyer, Halifax, Nova Scotia

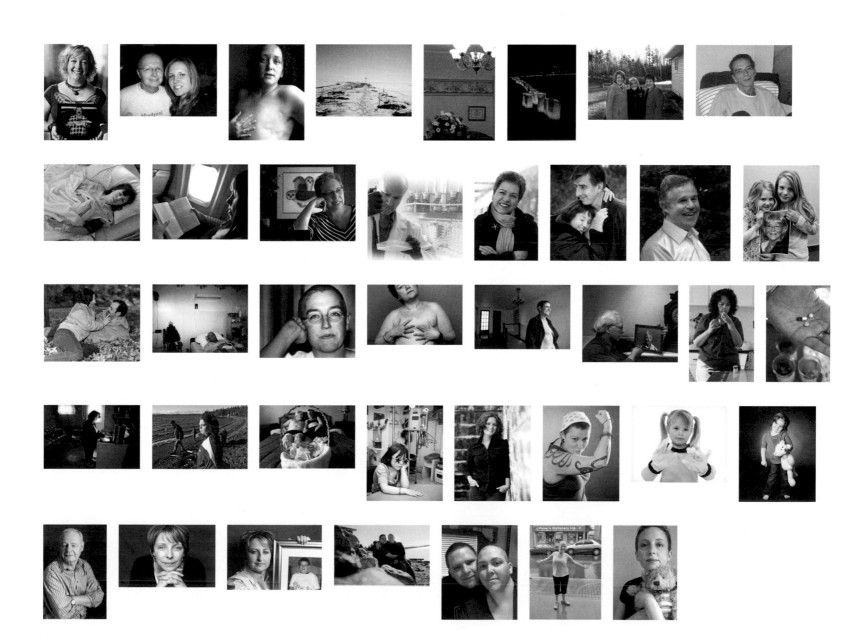

Schools

"Taking photographs for the project changed my outlook on cancer:

I developed hope for the future."

Briar Tedesco

James

James Ji, whose grandfather passed away from cancer. James remembers that it was raining on the day of his grandfather's funeral, and that mourners were holding black umbrellas. Rainy days remind him of that day and his grandfather.

Photographer
Seung Jae Lee
Ridley College
St.Catharines, Ontario

Keely

Keely's photo of a girl dancing in a field symbolizes the search for the cure for cancer and the hope that we are close to finding it. Keely says, "It also symbolizes the hope that we all carry in our hearts that the people suffering from cancer will be cured. The girls are jumping for joy and hope."

Photographer
Keely Maynard
St.Mildred's-Lightbourn
School, Oakville, Ontario

Keith and Hanna

Hanna Liscai with her hero, grandfather Keith Ford. Keith was diagnosed with lung cancer in 2003. Three years later the cancer had spread throughout his body, and soon after he passed away. "Luckily, he lived two years longer than expected, and he was always happy," says Hanna.

Photographer
Hanna Liscai
Matthews Hall School
London, Ontario

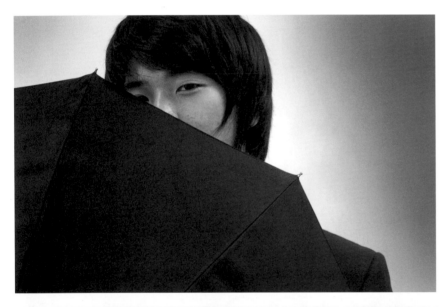

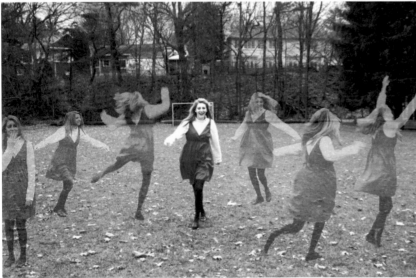

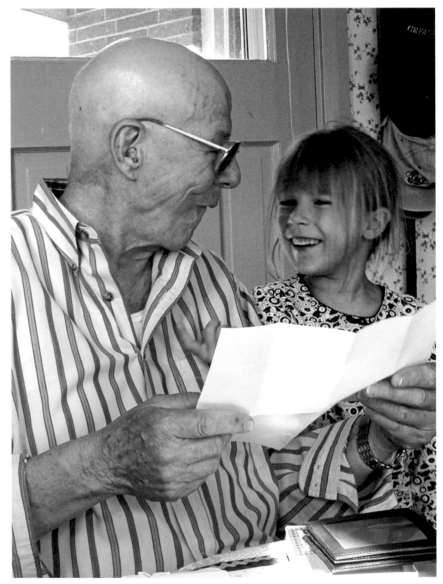

Vanessa

Photographer Vanessa French had classmates wear pink T-shirts and lie down in a field in the shape of a ribbon. Vanessa says, "I called my picture 'Save a Life,' because if we all stand together and make donations to breast cancer funds, we can all save a life. We need to find a cure for this disease."

Photographer
Vanessa French
Matthews Hall School
London, Ontario

Tess

Photographer Tess's pointe shoes from when she danced ballet. Her dance teacher, Miss Rebecca, was diagnosed with breast cancer in 2002. She recovered fully after chemotherapy and is back teaching.

Photographer
Tess Cowherd
Ridley College
St. Catharines, Ontario

James

Photographer Alana's father, James Lake, on a family vacation in Italy. James was diagnosed with prostate cancer in 2006, at age 56. Thanks to an early diagnosis and a successful prostatectomy, James is now well. Alana says, "Fortunately, my dad is a survivor and can continue to do the things he loves, like travel with us."

Photographer
Alana Ratcliff-Lake
St. Mildred's-Lightbourn
School, Oakville, Ontario

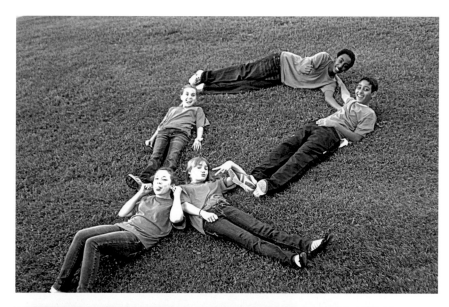

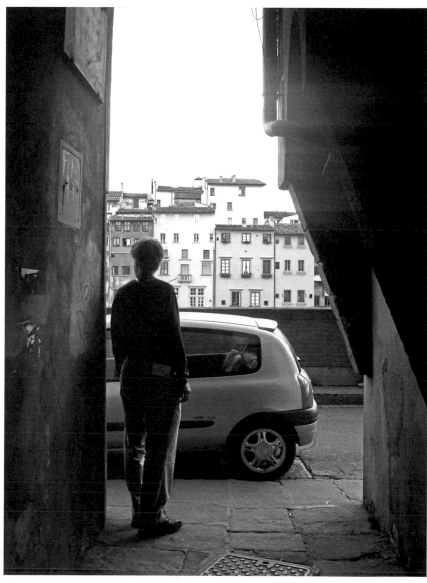

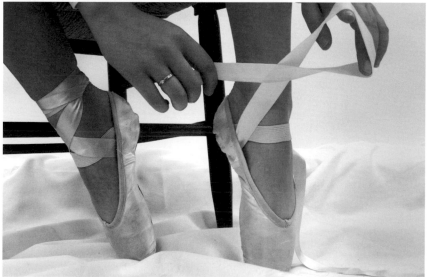

Andrew

Andrew Siu, staring at a photo of his grandmother, trying hard to remember her. "I hear stories about how much she loved me. It would be really nice if I could talk to her and share our thoughts together. I really don't have any memories of my grandmother, yet I miss her."

Photographer
Andrew Siu
Matthews Hall School
London, Ontario

Olivia

"Touching": Photographer Olivia Cullen's hand within a tracing of her grandfather Joseph Cullen's hand. Joseph had leukemia and underwent surgery and radiation before finally succumbing. Olivia says, "I traced his hand during his last days with us as a reminder of him. There is nothing more powerful than the human touch."

Photographer
Olivia Cullen
Matthews Hall School
London, Ontario

Braz for the Cause

Four decorated bras representing four years of the fundraising event, Braz for the Cause. Dr. Moira Cruickshank, who battled breast cancer herself, and her husband, Dr. David Massel, founded the event, which invites people to dress in themed bras, dance, eat, and share stories. Funds raised help women with breast cancer.

Photographer
Kristie Przewieda
Matthews Hall School
London, Ontario

Kyusik

This photograph represents the memories of times photographer Kyusik spent with his grandfather. He says, "We would sit on a bench in the park most of the day when I was living at his house and talk about my life. Now that he is in hospital, we cannot have the same talks. This photograph shows how I feel emptiness now that he is not near me."

Photographer
Kyusik Chung
Ridley College
St. Catharines, Ontario

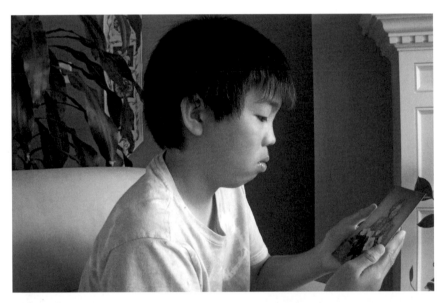

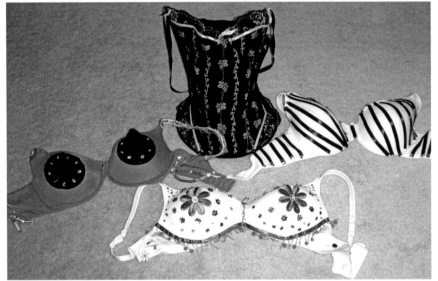

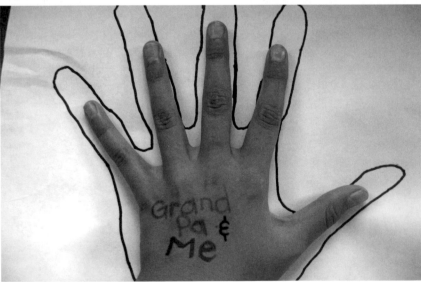

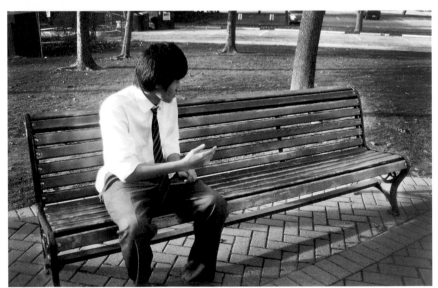

Elaine

Elaine Wong, a student at Ridley College, remembering her friend, Taylor Fung, who passed away from lung cancer. Elaine and Taylor would spend time talking and relaxing in coffee shops. Whenever Elaine visits coffee shops, she thinks about her friend.

Photographer
Enoch Ho
Ridley College
St. Catharines, Ontario

Rome

Photographer Rome's image demonstrates how cancer patients need support on their journey. Rome says, "People with cancer may feel lonely or isolated from others, with friends not visiting or calling. My photo represents how even the slightest touch can provide cancer patients with just the right amount of human contact and love to promote healing."

Photographer
Rome McCulloch
Greenwood College
Toronto, Ontario

Natalie

Natalie Whitney's photo represents the countdown in life faced by many cancer patients. Natalie says, "Cancer patients are not necessarily the only people who have cancer; their friends and family have it as well. Another year, another month, and another day are all blessings with this cruel disease."

Photographer
Natalie Whitney
Greenwood College
Toronto, Ontario

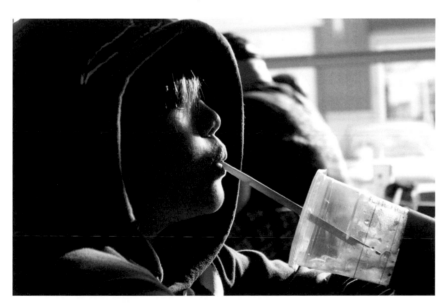

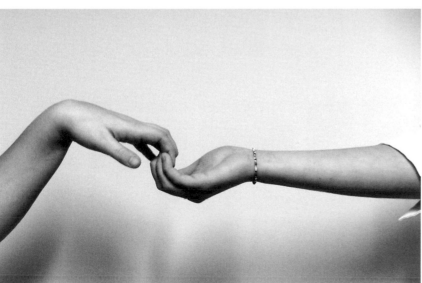

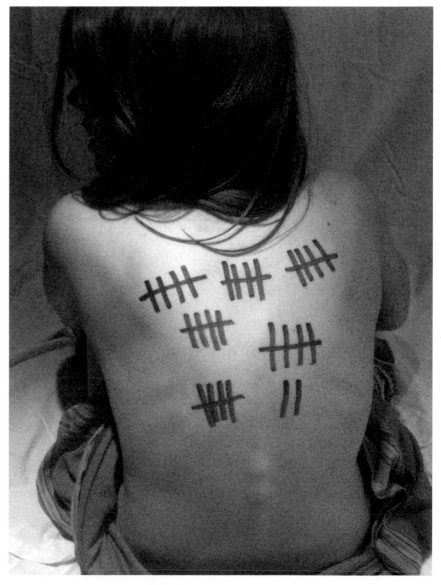

Row 1: Abigail Haines, St. Mildred's-Lightbourn School, Oakville, Ontario; Abigail Kaczmarek, St. Mildred's-Lightbourn School, Oakville, Ontario; Aitana Robinson, Matthews Hall School, London, Ontario; Alana Ratcliff-Lake (4–5), St. Mildred's-Lightbourn School, Oakville, Ontario; Alessandro Aquaviva, Matthews Hall School, London, Ontario; Alicia Banville, Ridley College, St. Catharines, Ontario; Alicia Pawluk, St. Michael's University School, Victoria, British Columbia

Row 2: Allen Chen, Ridley College, St. Catharines, Ontario; Allie Mitchell, Ridley College, St. Catharines, Ontario; Andrew Pickering, Matthews Hall School, London, Ontario; Anna Golubkova, Ridley College, St. Catharines, Ontario; Ashley Emerson, Matthews Hall School, London, Ontario; Avery McNair, Greenwood College, Toronto, Ontario; Beatriz Checa Gonzalez, Ridley College, St. Catharines, Ontario; Bemnet Dejene, Matthews Hall School, London, Ontario

Row 3: Ben Kulhanek, Ridley College, St. Catharines, Ontario; Brett Beauvais, Ridley College, St. Catharines, Ontario; Brett Beckley, Matthews Hall School, London, Ontario; Briar Tedesco (4–5), St. Mildred's-Lightbourn School, Oakville, Ontario; Cameron Sifton, Matthews Hall School, London, Ontario; Celine Caira, Greenwood College, Toronto, Ontario; Chelsea Fischer, Ridley College, St. Catharines, Ontario

Row 4: Cheryl Wong, Ridley College, St. Catharines, Ontario; Chloé Duggal, Matthews Hall School, London, Ontario; Chloe Hutcherson, Matthews Hall School, London, Ontario; Chris Massell, Matthews Hall School, London, Ontario; Clare Urquhart, Matthews Hall School, London, Ontario; Cole Gowanlock, Matthews Hall School, London, Ontario; Cole Van Alstine, Ridley College, St. Catharines, Ontario; Connor Velikonja, Matthews Hall School, London, Ontario

Row 5: Daniel Goodman, Matthews Hall School, London, Ontario; Danielle Tiger, Ridley College, St. Catharines, Ontario; David Dunbar, Matthews Hall School, London, Ontario; Denise Saad, Ridley College, St. Catharines, Ontario; Eden Church, Appleby College, Oakville, Ontario; Elliot Perera, Matthews Hall School, London, Ontario; Emma Hawkes, Appleby College, Oakville, Ontario; Emma Miller, Matthews Hall School, London, Ontario

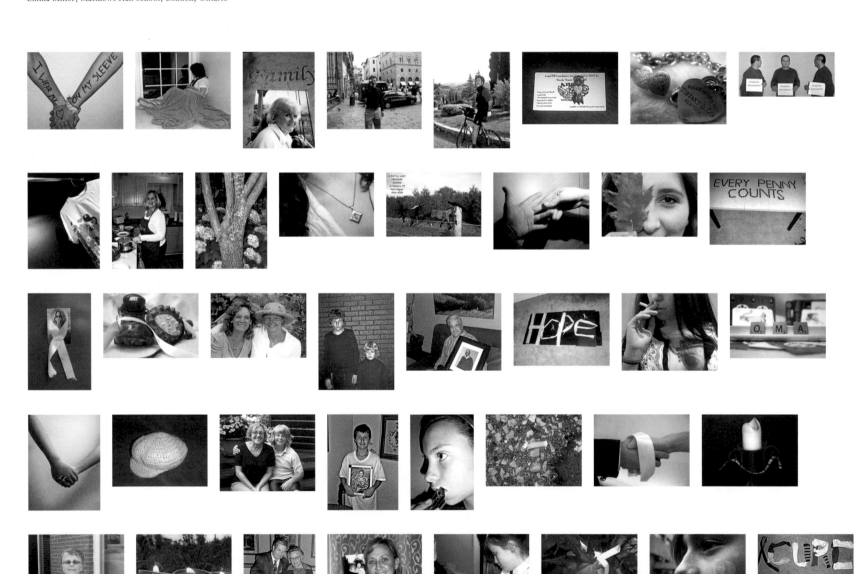

Row 1: Eryn Dickison (1–2), St. Mildred's-Lightbourn School, Oakville, Ontario; Eul Han, Matthews Hall School, London, Ontario; Fearghas Gundy, Ridley College, St. Catharines, Ontario; Gareth Ross, Matthews Hall School, London, Ontario; Garrett Riffal, Southridge School, Surrey, British Columbia; Georgina Evison, St. Mildred's-Lightbourn School, Oakville, Ontario; Grace Goble, Matthews Hall School, London, Ontario

Row 2: Graham Peck, Matthews Hall School, London, Ontario; Heidi Seguin, Ridley College, St. Catharines, Ontario; Hugh Kidd, Greenwood College, Toronto, Ontario; Hugh McHenry, Matthews Hall School, London, Ontario; Ilen Madhavji, Matthews Hall School, London, Ontario; Isabel Duchesne, Greenwood College, Toronto, Ontario; Isabella Bergagnini, St. Mildred's-Lightbourn School, Oakville, Ontario; Jaclyn Disney, Matthews Hall School, London, Ontario

Row 3: Jacqueline Olson, St. Mildred's-Lightbourn School, Oakville, Ontario; Jacqueline Toole, Greenwood College, Toronto, Ontario; James Spadafora, Matthews Hall School, London, Ontario; Jared Dodman, Ridley College, St. Catharines, Ontario; Jason Wallenburg, Greenwood College, Toronto, Ontario; Jennifer Halsall, St. Mildred's-Lightbourn School, Oakville, Ontario; Jenny Lee, Matthews Hall School, London, Ontario; Jessica Tucker, Matthews Hall School, London, Ontario

Row 4: Joelle Matthews (1–2), Greenwood College, Toronto, Ontario; John Hord, Matthews Hall School, London, Ontario; John Hughes, Greenwood College, Toronto, Ontario; John Lee, Matthews Hall School, London, Ontario; Joshua Bainbridge, Matthews Hall School, London, Ontario; Joshua deHoog, Matthews Hall School, London, Ontario; Joyce Chow, Appleby College, Oakville, Ontario

Row 5: Joyce Du (1–2), Appleby College, Oakville, Ontario; Kaylynn Purdy (3–4), St. Michael's University School, Victoria, British Columbia; Keely Maynard (5–6), St. Mildred's-Lightbourn School, Oakville, Ontario; Kennedy Velikonja, Matthews Hall School, London, Ontario; Kenzie Goodall, St. Mildred's-Lightbourn School, Oakville, Ontario

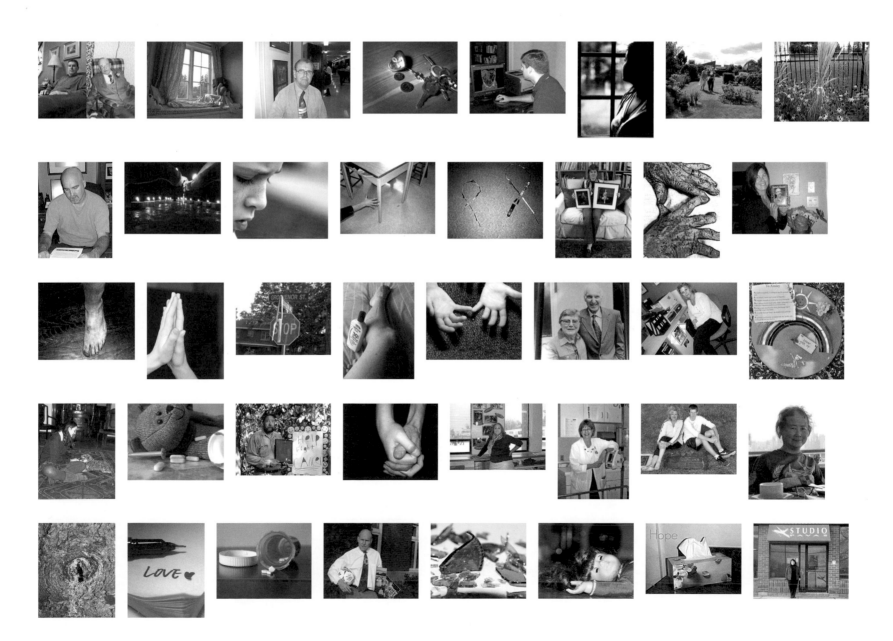

Row 1: Kiely Clarke, Matthews Hall School, London, Ontario; Kiersten Waugh, Matthews Hall School, London, Ontario; Larissa Pencak, St Mildred's-Lightbourn School, Oakville, Ontario; Luke Kadey (4–5), Greenwood College, Toronto, Ontario, Maddie Goodall (6–8), St. Mildred's-Lightbourn School, Oakville, Ontario

Row 2: Maddie Goodall (1–3), St. Mildred's-Lightbourn School, Oakville, Ontario; Madison Kennedy, Greenwood College, Toronto, Ontario; Maëlle Marchand; St. Mildred's-Lightbourn School, Oakville, Ontario; Mariska Batohi, Matthews Hall School, London, Ontario; Marius Froehlich, Ridley College, St. Catharines, Ontario; Mary-Laure New, Matthews Hall School, London, Ontario

Row 3: Maryann Watson, St. Michael's University School, Victoria, British Columbia; Mason Hermann, Matthews Hall School, London, Ontario; Matthew Wiseman, Matthews Hall School, London, Ontario; Matthew Pizzo, Ridley College, St. Catharines, Ontario; Meaghan Gallant (5–6), St. Mildred's-Lightbourn School, Oakville, Ontario; Meesam Naqvi, Ridley College, St. Catharines, Ontario; Meg Squires, Ridley College, St. Catharines, Ontario

Row 4: Megan Miller, Ridley College, St. Catharines, Ontario; Micaelyn Mann, Matthews Hall School, London, Ontario; Micayla Miller, Matthews Hall School, London, Ontario; Min Ha Kim, St. Michael's University School, Victoria, British Columbia, Miranda Rogovein, Greenwood College, Toronto, Ontario; Moises Cohen Saba, Ridley College, St. Catharines, Ontario; Molly Betker, Matthews Hall School, London, Ontario; Monica Scrocchi, Matthews Hall School, London, Ontario

Row 5: Morgan Kaufman, Greenwood College, Toronto, Ontario; Natalie Shewan, Matthews Hall School, London, Ontario; Nicholas Haines, Matthews Hall School, London, Ontario; Nicole Clydesdale, St. Mildred's-Lightbourn School, Oakville, Ontario, Nikhil Taneja, Matthews Hall School, London, Ontario; Olamiposi Akinsooto, Matthews Hall School, London, Ontario; Owen Thompson, Matthews Hall School, London, Ontario; Paisley Shannon, Matthews Hall School, London, Ontario

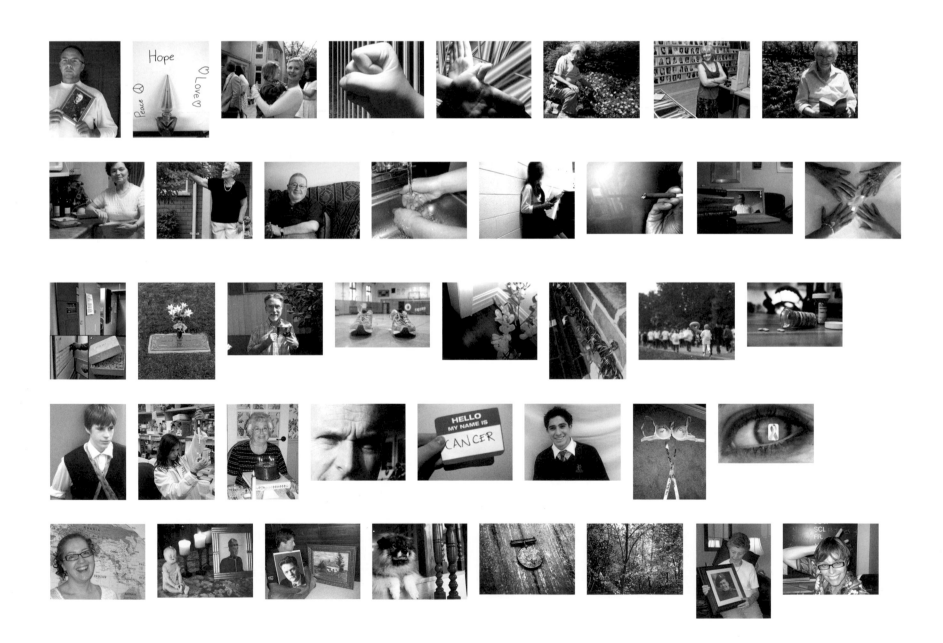

Row 1: Paul Kim, Matthews Hall School, London, Ontario; Peter Park, Ridley College, St. Catharines, Ontario; Rachael Aragona (3–4), St. Mildred's-Lightbourn School, Oakville, Ontario, Robin Winship, St. Mildred's-Lightbourn School, Oakville, Ontario; Sam Carlton, Greenwood College, Toronto, Ontario; Samuel Gerofsky, Matthews Hall School, London, Ontario; Samantha Ambrosie, St. Mildred's-Lightbourn School, Oakville, Ontario

Row 2: Samantha Ambrosie, St. Mildred's-Lightbourn School, Oakville, Ontario; Samuel Weinberger, Matthews Hall School, London, Ontario; Sarah Asper, Greenwood College, Toronto, Ontario; Sarah Brymer, Matthews Hall School, London, Ontario; Sarah Burns, Matthews Hall School, London, Ontario; Sarah Krause, Matthews Hall School, London, Ontario; Sarah Mentner, Ridley College, St. Catharines, Ontario; Sean Kim, Matthews Hall School, London, Ontario

Row 3: Sean Luke, Matthews Hall School, London, Ontario; Sonja Drosdowech, Matthews Hall School, London, Ontario; Spencer Shannon, Matthews Hall School, London, Ontario; Stephanie Li, Matthews Hall School, London, Ontario; Stephanie Singeris, Matthews Hall School, London, Ontario; Stephanie Skanes, Matthews Hall School, London, Ontario; Stephany Guillen, Ridley College, St. Catharines, Ontario; Svea Kolbe, Matthews Hall School, London, Ontario

Row 4: Sydney DiFruscia, Matthews Hall School, London, Ontario; Talia Thomson, Appleby College, Oakville, Ontario io; Tessa Peerless, Matthews Hall School, London, Ontario; Tiffany Ma, Matthews Hall School, London, Ontario; Tom McHenry, Matthews Hall School, London, Ontario; Travis DeWolf (6–7), St. Mildred's-Lightbourn School, Oakville, Ontario; Tygre Patchell-Evans, Matthews Hall School, London, Ontario

Row 5: Tyler Waugh, Matthews Hall School, London, Ontario; Victoria Sanderson, Matthews Hall School, London, Ontario; Vlad Beliaev, Matthews Hall School, London, Ontario; Wendy Liu, Ridley College, St. Catharines, Ontario; Weston Crawford, Matthews Hall School, London, Ontario; Will Luke, Matthews Hall School, London, Ontario; Wincy Li, Ridley College, St. Catharines, Ontario; Zohra Bhimani, Matthews Hall School, London, Ontario

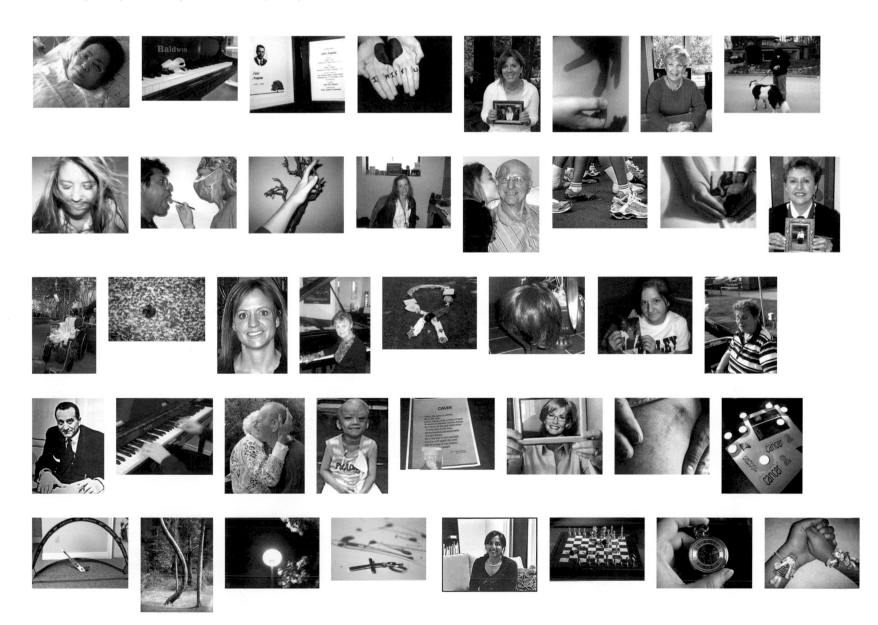

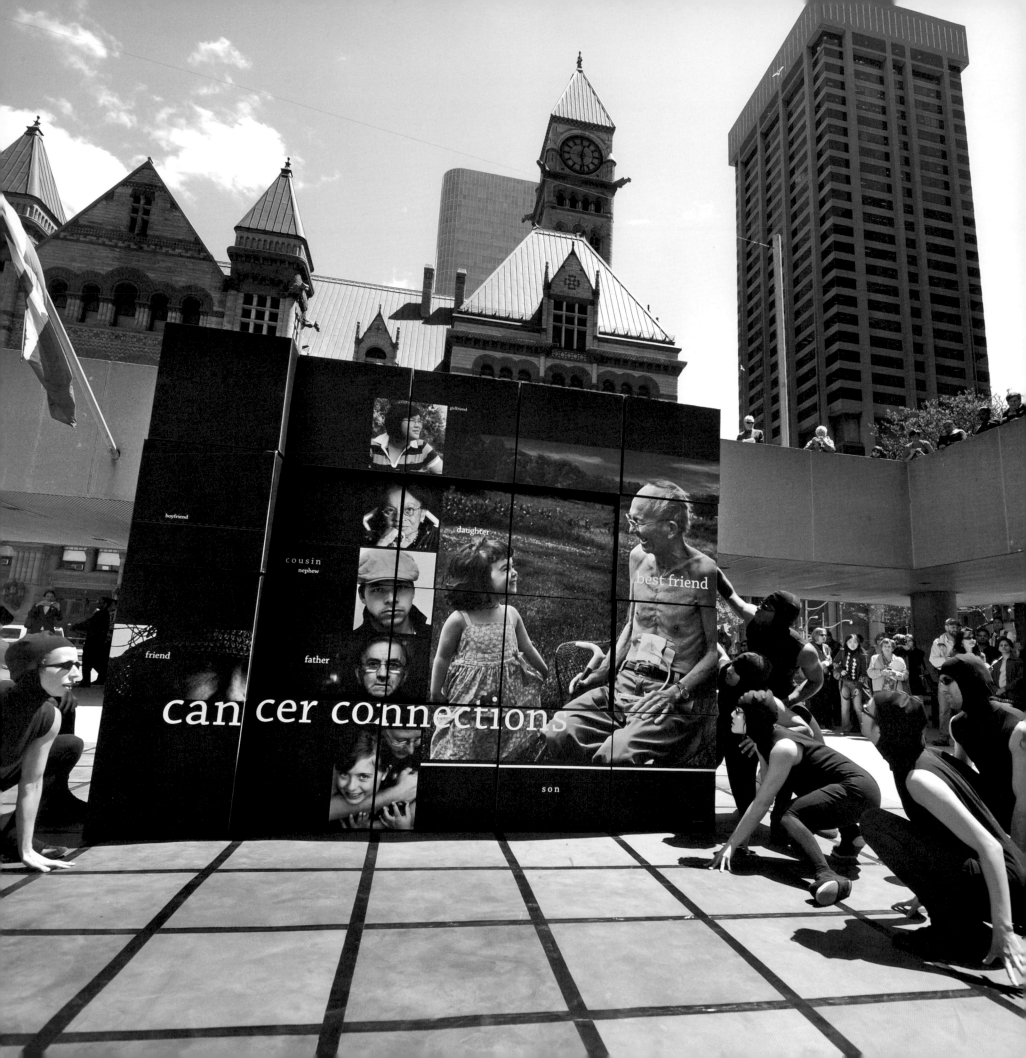

Toronto, Ontario

Cancer Connections' inaugural exhibition opened at City Hall, Nathan Phillips Square in Toronto on May 20, 2008. Dance troupe AntiGravity entertained the crowd after the opening speeches, building a *Cancer Connections* wall.

Photographer
Aaron Vincent Elkaim

The *Cancer Connections* Tour

When we launched the *Cancer Connections* exhibition, our aim was to reach as many Canadians as possible. And so we produced PhotoSensitive's most ambitious project yet: a touring, ever-expanding, bilingual show displayed in outdoor public areas that would visit every single province.

The exhibition opened at Toronto's Nathan Phillips Square on May 20, 2008, with 270 photos on display. Hundreds of people attended the celebration, which was opened by Toronto mayor David Miller. Over 100 of the photographers and subjects attended, beginning a trend that would continue in every city visited over the next two years.

After Toronto, the exhibition went to Charlottetown and then travelled across Canada. Each city brought more submissions and the number of photos on display grew with each stop.

This was the first time in PhotoSensitive's 20-year history that an exhibition was designed specifically for the outdoors. It had to be able to withstand blazing sun, rain, hail, snow, and gale-force winds. The structures and photo panels, when installed, were themselves a work of art and fitted in beautifully with their surroundings.

Auspiciously, *Cancer Connections* was blessed with fair weather for every one of its openings. In many places, like Newfoundland and Winnipeg, the weather was terrible before and after the launch but clouds dispersed in time for the opening and crowds enjoyed the ceremony under clear skies.

By the time *Cancer Connections* arrived in Ottawa for its finale on June 1, 2010, it had travelled over 17,000 kilometres, visited every province, grown to an online gallery of 1,000 photos, and been seen by hundreds of thousands of people.

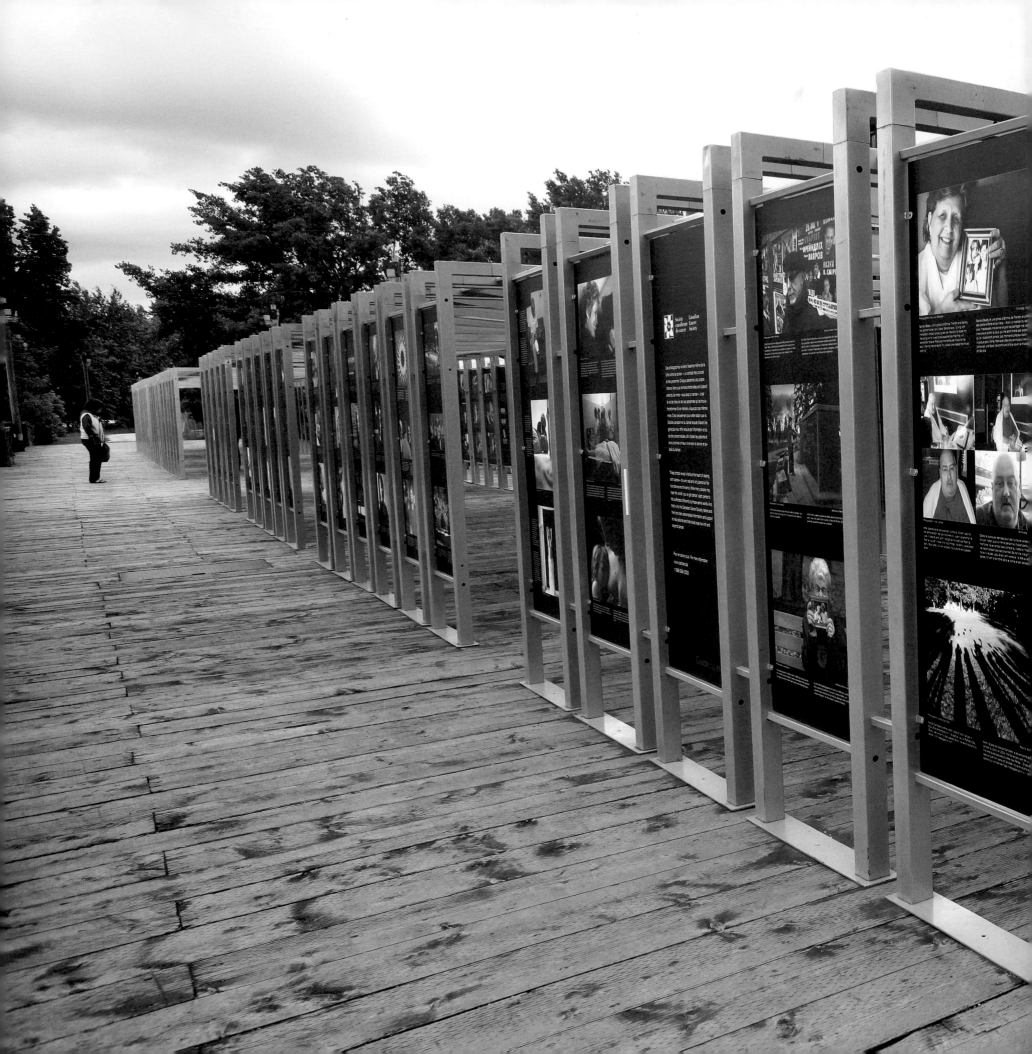

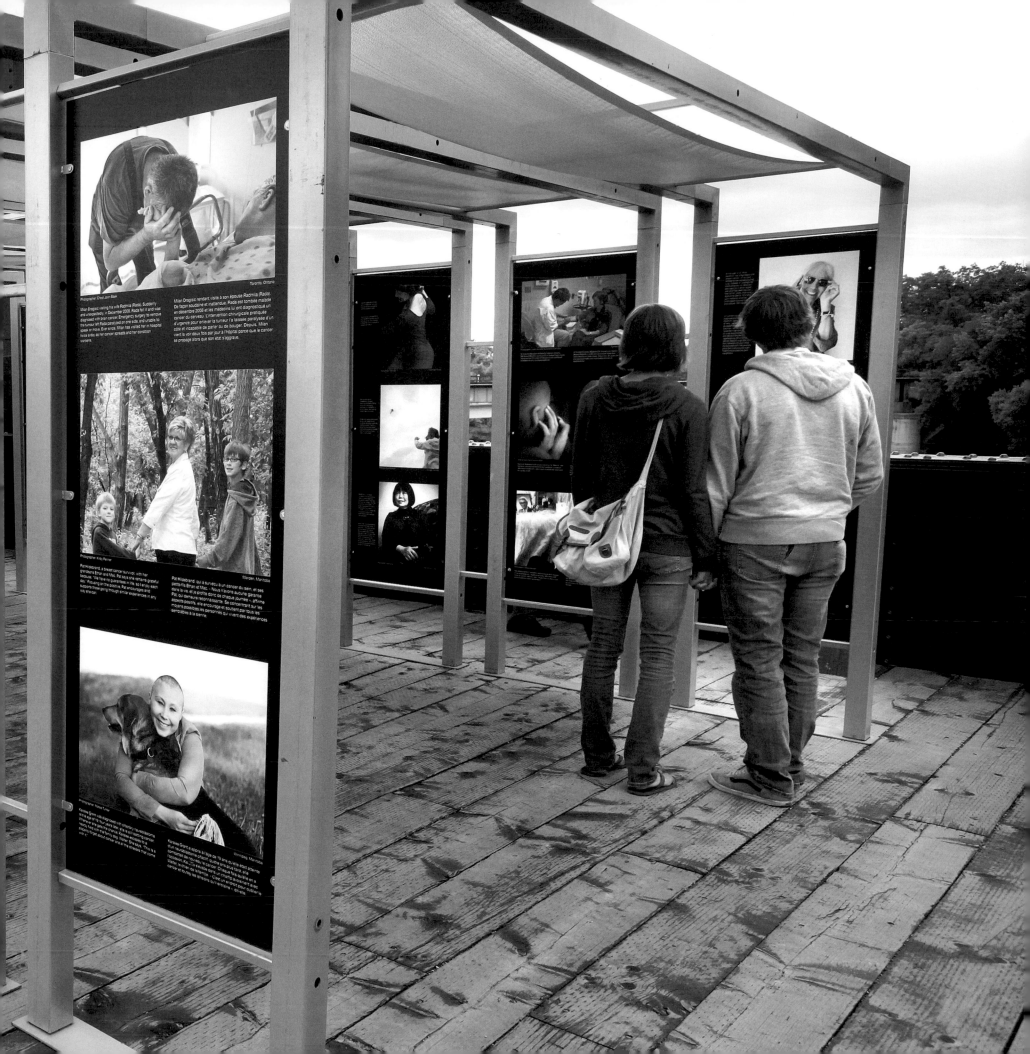

Previous

Winnipeg, Manitoba

Cancer Connections was displayed across The Forks Historic Rail Bridge in downtown Winnipeg in July 2009. The Forks, which overlooks the spot where the Assiniboine and Red rivers meet, has been a meeting place for 6,000 years, receives over 4 million visitors a year, and provided the perfect location for the exhibition.

Photographer
Andrew Stawicki

Halifax, Nova Scotia

PhotoSensitive project coordinator, James Burns, films *Cancer Connections* subject Ryan Joudrey next to his photo, during the Halifax opening at Dalhousie University, in September 2009. PhotoSensitive photographed and filmed hundreds of subjects and photographers at 11 opening ceremonies for inclusion on the *Cancer Connections* website.

Photographer
Shari Tucker

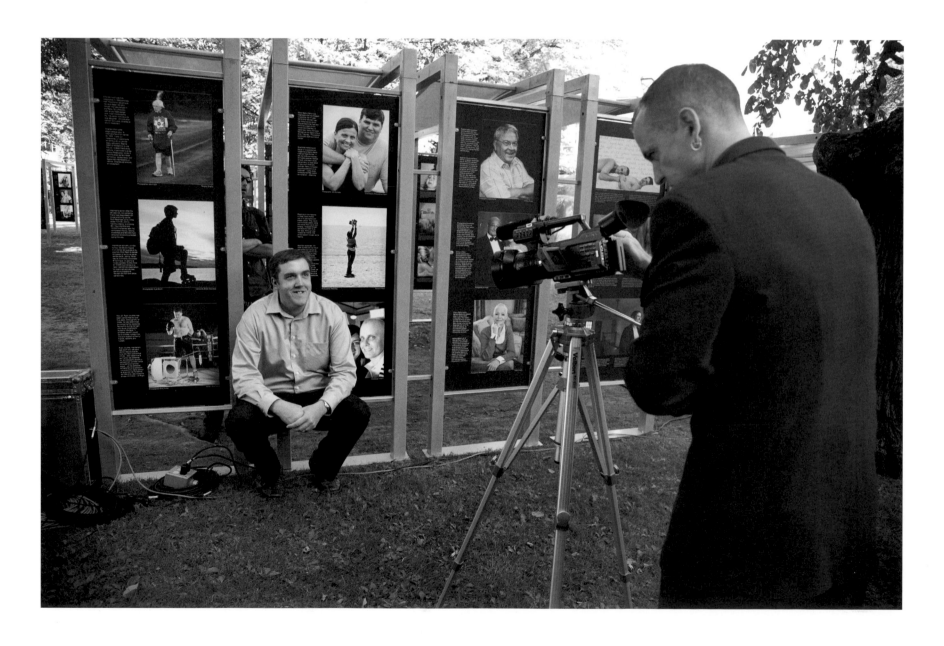

Ottawa, Ontario

Speakers, subjects, and photographers gathered to celebrate *Cancer Connections'* finale opening ceremony in Ottawa at Major's Hill Park in June 2010.

Photographer
Jon Currie

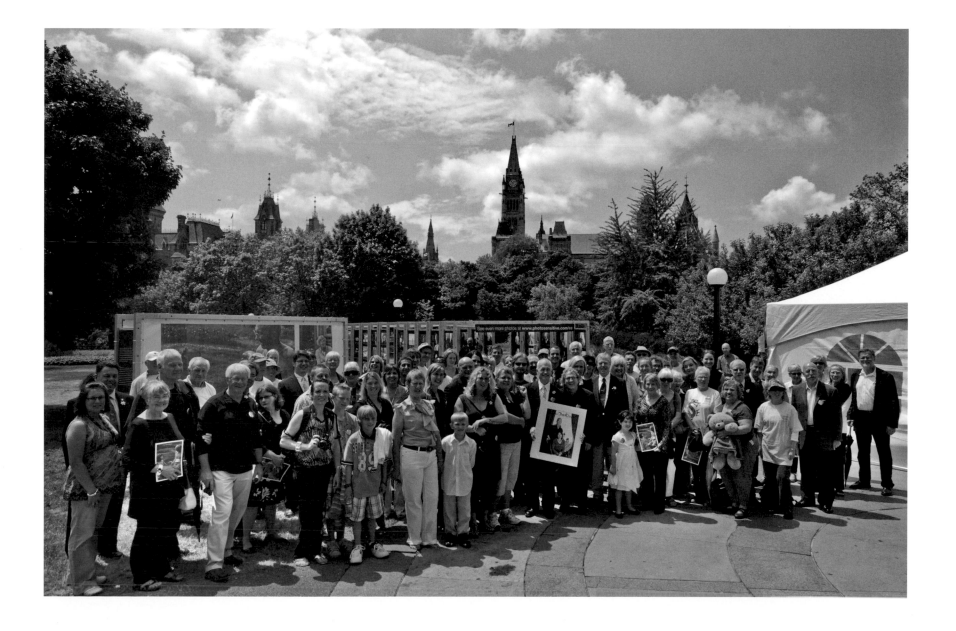

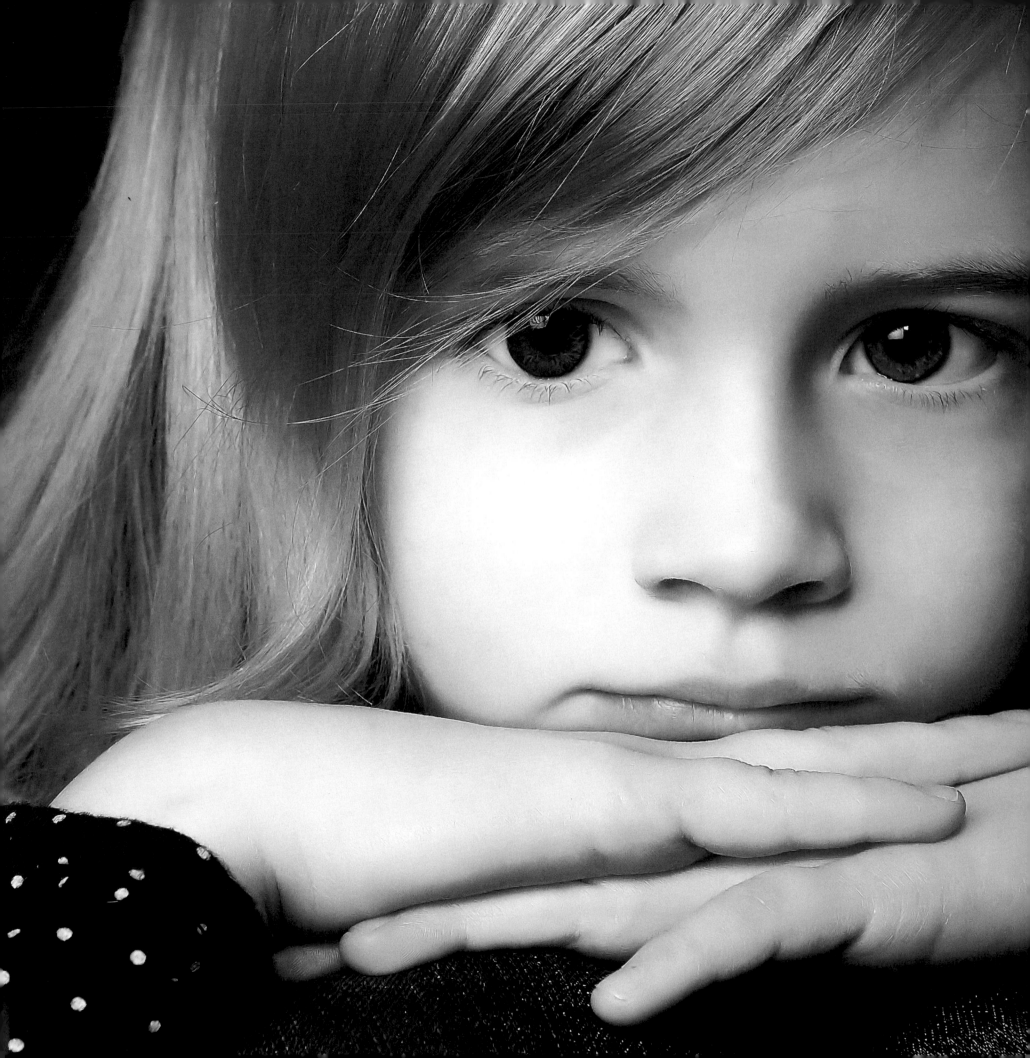

Over

Makenna

Five-year-old Makenna was diagnosed with bilateral retinoblastoma (eye cancer) at three months old. She lost her right eye to cancer and underwent chemotherapy, laser therapy and cryo-therapy to save her left eye. Makenna has been cancer-free since June 2005.

Photographer
Alex Mackie
Stittsville, Ontario

Join the Fight

The Canadian Cancer Society's display at the Canada Blooms exhibition in Toronto in March 2010 included a "Join the Fight" wall. Visitors were invited to write a message related to cancer. By the end of the week, the wall was filled with messages of support, hope, and defiance.

Photographer
Hugh Wesley
Toronto, Ontario

Acknowledgements

Ideas are powerful, but without the support of friends and colleagues to make them happen, they are just ideas. In producing *Cancer Connections*, the book and the exhibition, PhotoSensitive has been fortunate to have the extraordinary support of some great people.

We are ever grateful to the generous and amazing photographers who gave their time, energy, and creativity to show the life and spirit of people touched by cancer.

To all the people who so generously allowed our cameras to capture some of the most intimate moments of their lives, thank you on behalf of so many.

A huge thanks to our sponsors, whose much appreciated contributions were invaluable in putting together this book: Epson Canada and Our Kids Publications.

Our deep appreciation to our *Cancer Connections* partners; the Canadian Cancer Society, which was crucial in ensuring a successful, nationwide exhibition, and to all of the provincial divisions of the Canadian Cancer Society which secured excellent locations for the exhibition, guaranteeing that thousands of people in their province got to see the show.

We are grateful to our presenting sponsor, JPMorgan Chase, which provided the financial support that allowed the exhibition to travel across the country.

Our thanks to all of you.

PhotoSensitive

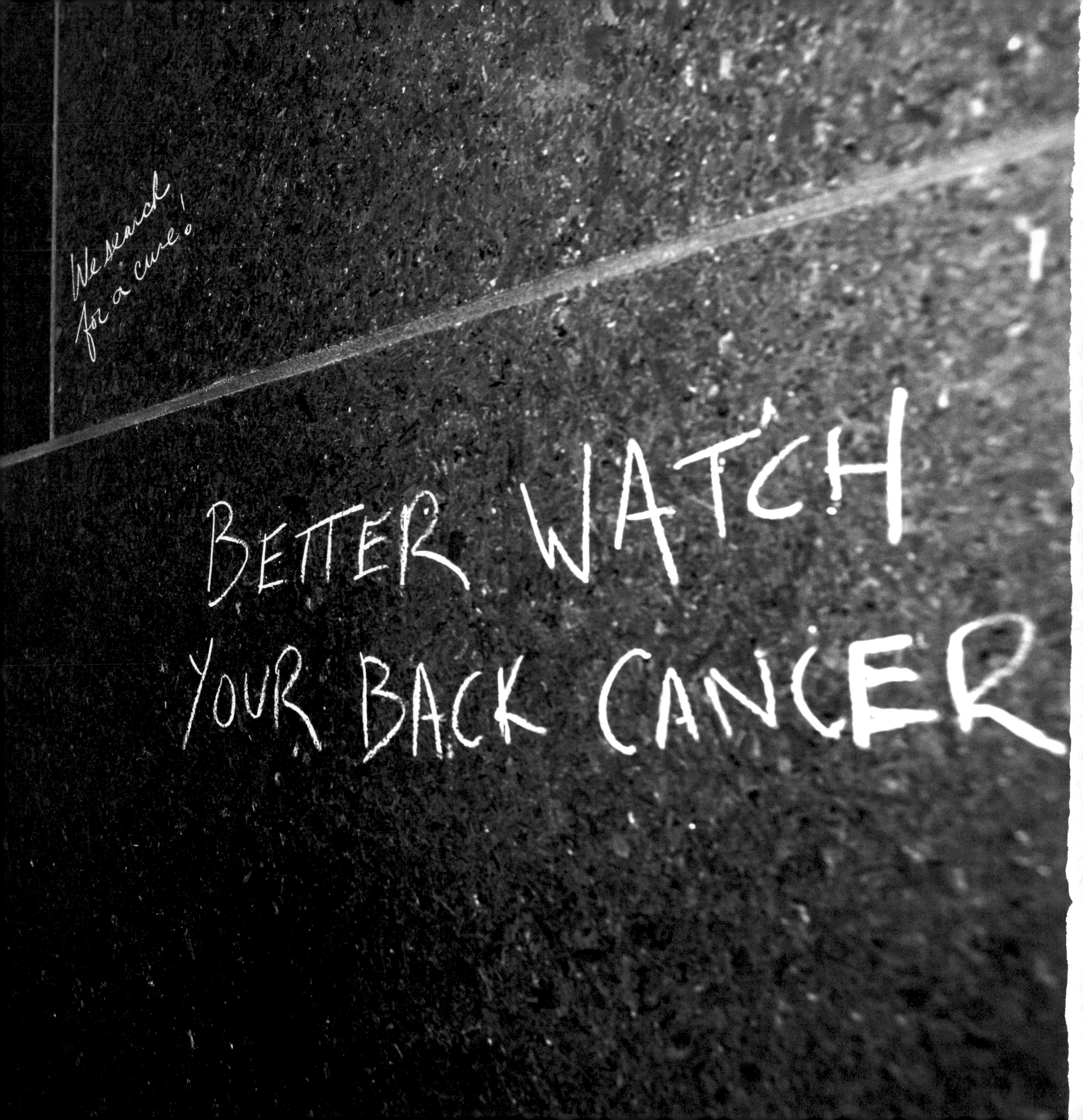
We search for a cure!
BETTER WATCH YOUR BACK CANCER